LIBRARIES NI
WITHDRAWN FROM STOCK
D0270351

About the Authors

Dr Roger Henderson was born in 1960 and raised in Whitehaven, Cumbria. He qualified as a doctor from St Bartholomew's Hospital, London in 1985 and as a general practitioner in 1990. He entered the media world in 1995, and is now one of the UK's most respected media medics, writing regular columns for national newspapers and magazines. He is also a popular lecturer and after-dinner motivational speaker on a wide range of health-related topics and his medical responsibilities include being the senior partner of a six doctor general practice, running a main surgery and two busy branch surgeries. Married to a doctor, and with three teenage children, his spare time is spent thinking about how nice it would be to have some spare time.

Matthew M. F. Miller is a dad to one, an uncle to ten, and a 'father' to anyone who will listen to his countless nuggets of unsolicited advice. Author of the book *Maybe Baby: An Infertile Love Story,* Matthew is a graduate of the University of Southern California's Master of Professional Writing program. Matthew lives in Chicago where he is a full-time work-at-home dad, providing childcare for his daughter while working as the health-and-wellness editor for a national newspaper syndicate. In his spare time (because there's just so much of that!), Matthew is a musician, runner, tennis enthusiast and baker.

Sharon Perkins has never been a dad, but she's had lots of experience on the mum side of parenting, with five children and three grandchildren. Almost 25 years as a registered nurse in fertility, labour and delivery, and neonatal intensive care have also taught her a thing or two about pregnancy and babies. Sharon lives in New Jersey with her husband but would live in Disney World if it were legal. The opportunity to write about what she does for a living has been a dream come true.

LIBRARIES NI	
C900233036	
Bertrams	02/03/2012
618.20081	£10.99
LURGRP	

Dedication

From Roger: For Becky, Douglas, Sarah and Jack. Always.

From Matt: Whether writing this book, watching tennis, or taking a nap, I am inspired, awed and grateful for the love and support of my wife, Constance, and our beautiful daughter, Nola. Thank you for a charmed life.

From Sharon: This book is dedicated to my three grandchildren, Matthew, Emma and Jessica, who keep me current on what's going on in the world of kids.

Authors' Acknowledgments

From Matt: Writing about family takes a deep, rich understanding of what it means to be a good person, and I am grateful to my mom, dad, sisters, nieces, and nephews for teaching me how to be one. Also, a very special thanks to my favorite doula, Holly Barhamand, for teaching and empowering me to explore and educate myself about what childbirth means to me. As this is my first *For Dummies* tome, I am particularly grateful to the folks at Wiley, but also to Sharon herself. She took me under her wing and made this one of the most rewarding, fun experiences of my writing career. To my agent, Grace Freedson, you are a joy to work with and I look forward to the next amazing opportunity you bring my way. Finally, thank you to my wife and, most importantly, to our daughter, an IVF baby born after nearly three years of waiting. And although we waited a long time for you, every day since your birth has been counted among the best of my life.

From Sharon: Wiley took a chance on me with my first book, Fertility For Dummies, almost ten years ago, and I've been extremely grateful ever since. In particular, Lindsay Lefevere, Erin Mooney, Chrissy Guthrie, and Caitie Copple have been the usual pleasure to work with throughout this book's creation. Matt Miller has been the easiest coauthor ever! From day one, our writing styles meshed, and this book just flowed. Thanks, Matt, for making this a piece of cake. And, last but not least, I thank my family for giving me so much raw material to work with over the years!

Publisher's Acknowledgments

We're proud of this book; please send us your comments at http://dummies.custhelp.com. For other comments, please contact our Customer Care Department within the U.S. at 877-762-2974, outside the U.S. at 317-572-3993, or fax 317-572-4002.

Some of the people who helped bring this book to market include the following:

Acquisitions, Editorial, and Vertical Websites

Project Editor: Simon Bell
(Previous Edition: Christina Guthrie)

Acquisitions Editor: Mike Baker

Copy Editor: Kate O' Leary

Technical Reviewer: Dr Klare Davis

Assistant Editor: Ben Kemble

Production Manager: Daniel Mersey

Publisher: David Palmer

Cover Photos: © iStock /
Agnieszka Szymczak

Cartoons: Ed McLachlan

Composition Services

Project Coordinator: Kristie Rees

Layout and Graphics: Lavonne Roberts,
Corrie Socolovitch

Proofreader: Lauren Mandelbaum

Indexer: Estalita Slivoskey

Publishing and Editorial for Consumer Dummies

    Kathleen Nebenhaus, Vice President and Executive Publisher

    Kristin Ferguson-Wagstaffe, Product Development Director

    Ensley Eikenburg, Associate Publisher, Travel

    Kelly Regan, Editorial Director, Travel

Publishing for Technology Dummies

    Andy Cummings, Vice President and Publisher

Composition Services

    Debbie Stailey, Director of Composition Services

Contents at a Glance

Table of Contents

Introduction

● ●

*W*elcome to impending fatherhood! Being a dad is better than you can ever imagine and far less scary than you're probably believing it to be. One of the main reasons we wrote this book was to empower men to get actively involved in every aspect of the childbirth process, as well as the care, feeding and loving of newborns. Most dads-to-be have only a dim idea of what parenthood is going to be like, and their excitement mixes liberally with sheer terror and trepidation. We hope this book spares you some of that fear and trepidation by giving you the knowledge you need to feel confident.

Traditionally, men have been removed from the processes of pregnancy, labour and delivery, and raising children. On TV, fathers have long been portrayed as emotionally distant, bumbling fools incapable of changing nappies, getting kids to go to bed or handling any of the routine tasks that mothers seem to do with ease. In reality, today's dad is confident, capable and totally in love with his children – and not afraid to let it show. Not that it all comes easily and naturally. Learning how to support your pregnant partner and, subsequently, to care for a newborn, takes time, effort and education.

Most men in the world will become fathers at some point, and most will enter the experience without much knowledge of how babies develop, how to be a supportive partner or what their role should be in the process. But not you. The savvy readers of this book will be prepared for just about anything – and will know exactly what it takes to be an equal partner on the pregnancy (and parenting) journey.

About This Book

This book answers all the burning questions you have about the impact your partner's pregnancy will have on your life. We tell you how your sex life will change, because we know that's pretty important. But we also explain everything you ever wanted to know about how a foetus develops, what living with a pregnant woman is like and how your wallet will be hit by adding a new member (or members) to your family.

We also delve a little into what to expect in the first six months or so after the baby arrives. We walk you through the ins and outs of feeding, changing nappies, dealing with common illnesses and emergencies, and how to stay sane and true to yourself through it all.

In short, you'll close this book feeling completely prepared for fatherhood. You won't be, because no one ever is, but you'll at least feel like you are until the baby comes.

Conventions Used in This Book

Following are a few conventions we used when writing this book:

- ✔ We don't know if your baby is a boy or girl – you may not even know that yourself. So we use *he* and *she* in alternate chapters.

- ✔ Because we also don't know if your medical practitioner is a doctor or midwife, or a paediatrician or nurse practitioner, we use the term *medical practitioner* when we talk about anyone medical.

- ✔ We call your partner your partner, because that's what she is, in every sense.

- ✔ We use an *italic* font to highlight new terms, and we follow them up with a clear definition.

- ✔ We use a **bold** font to indicate keywords or the actions in numbered steps.

- ✔ We use `Monofont` for web addresses.

What You're Not to Read

If you decide this book is too long, you may decide to skip some of it and thus want to know what's not very important. Naturally, we think every word we've written is not only essential but brilliant, so we're the wrong people to ask. However, information marked with the Technical Stuff icon may be more than you want to have to think about. Information marked with this icon is certainly interesting and helpful, but skipping it won't impede your understanding of the topic in the slightest.

Also, we've included sidebars throughout the book (look for grey-shaded boxes) that often contain interesting but non-essential information and personal stories, and we give you permission to skip them if you really have to.

If your partner is already pregnant, congratulations! That means you can skip Chapter 2, which discusses conception. And we hope everyone will be able to skip reading Chapter 12, which discusses problems that can come up after delivery. However, you may still want to skim this one so you'll know where to turn in the unfortunate event of complications.

Foolish Assumptions

If you picked up this book, we assume you fall into at least one of the following categories:

✔ You don't know much about pregnancy.

✔ You're an expectant dad.

✔ You're hoping to become an expectant dad.

✔ You're already a father but are looking to learn new tricks for the next go-round.

✔ You know an expectant dad and would like to get into his head and understand why he's behaving the way he is.

Expectant dads are often the forgotten partner in the new family-to-be, and they need all the understanding they can get.

How This Book Is Organised

This book starts with the process of getting pregnant and ends with practical information on day-to-day dad stuff. However, we know you may not be interested in reading about the journey straight through from beginning to end. So feel free to start wherever you want. If tomorrow is your first ultrasound appointment, jump right into that section so you know what to expect. If your partner isn't pregnant yet but you want to read about labour, go right ahead. Every chapter of this book is modular, which means you can understand it without reading other chapters first.

Part 1: So You Want to Be a Dad . . .

Becoming a dad is one of the most exciting times of a man's life, but that doesn't mean you don't also have concerns and questions. This part dives into the normal fears and frustrations associated with deciding to start a family and the actual process of getting pregnant – and no, you don't already know it all!

Part II: Great Expectations: Nine Months and Counting

Your partner may be the one who's pregnant, but you're in it for the ride, too. From morning sickness to labour, we tell you exactly what happens during pregnancy, from your perspective as well as hers and the baby's. We also talk about the fun stuff, like naming the baby, and the not fun stuff, like potential health issues for mum and baby. We also give you an overview of birthing options so you can talk knowledgeably with your partner about what she wants to do.

Part III: Game Time! Labour, Delivery and Baby's Homecoming

No one ever said labour and delivery are fun, but they are interesting, and you have a lot to learn if you want to win the supportive partner of the year award. This part covers everything about actually having the baby, from the first contraction to the first all-night crying session – which just may come from an exhausted parent, not the baby!

Part IV: A Dad's Guide to Worrying

This part touches on all the things that keep you up at night worrying after the baby is born. We discuss possible post-delivery issues such as congenital defects and postpartum depression as well as baby's inevitable illnesses. If your worries are more monetary, we also advise you on handling your money now that you have an expensive new baby and planning for your family's financial security. We also help you stay sane and happy with suggestions for managing your time so that you don't let the new baby take over your life.

Part V: The Part of Tens

The Part of Tens is just fun. We touch on how to be both a super dad and a super partner. We also talk about what it's like to be a stay-at-home dad.

Icons Used in This Book

Icons are another handy tool you can use as you work your way through this book. If you find the tips really helpful, for instance, you can skim through and search for that icon. Conversely, when you see a Technical Stuff icon, you can know that you can skip that information (though it's certainly worth the extra time, if you have it).

Following is a rundown of the icons we use in this book:

The Remember icon sits next to information we hope stays in your head for more than two minutes.

Technical Stuff goes into more detail than you really need to understand the facts, but you may find it interesting if you're an especially curious type.

The Tip icon gives helpful insider info that you may take years to learn on your own.

Whenever we use a Warning icon, you'd better sit up and take notice, because not heeding our warning could entail big problems for you or your loved ones.

Where to Go from Here

This is where we tell you to get on with it and read the book.

Although you can start absolutely any place and get the benefit of our expertise, if your partner isn't yet pregnant or is newly pregnant, we suggest starting at the beginning and reading right on through. Doing so will calm your nerves, we promise.

If you're the last-minute type of guy and you're reading this book just a few months (or weeks!) before the impending birth, you can certainly skip the first trimester stuff (at least this time around) and start wherever makes the most sense for you.

And if you got this book at the beginning of the pregnancy but never got around to opening it until now, when baby has her first case of sniffles, that's okay too – we still have plenty of valuable information for you. Pregnancy is the start of the adventure, but the fun continues long after.

Part I
So You Want to Be a Dad . . .

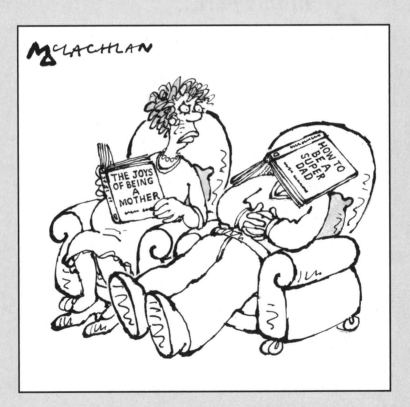

In this part...

Chances are, the road to fatherhood wasn't something you dwelled on much in your earlier years. When you decide to begin a family, though, exciting thoughts about conception alternate with fears of not being a good dad and concerns about money, time, and a brand-new way of life. In this part we look at the doubts and worries that consume every new dad-to-be and explain the mechanics of getting pregnant. You may think this is one area where you need no help, but many couples find getting pregnant a frustrating struggle, and even those who don't can benefit from a refresher course on conception.

Chapter 1

Fatherhood: A Glorious, Scary, Mind-Boggling and Amazing Experience

In This Chapter

▶ Exploring what it means to be a father today

▶ Understanding what will change in your life

▶ Facing the decision of whether to have a baby

▶ Looking down the long road ahead

Apparently, congratulations are in order: either you're going to be a father sometime within the next nine months or you're in the planning stages of becoming a dad. Either way, you've come to the right place. You'll face no bigger life decision than choosing to become a parent (and no bigger jolt than being told baby is coming if you didn't expect it!), and the best gift you can give to your soon-to-be child is confidence. And the only way to feel confident before you've ever been a parent is to get yourself prepared for the unknown journey that lies ahead.

Perhaps you've already been floored by equal doses of joy and fear, which is a good sign that you both recognise the magnitude of the change and are up for the challenge of fatherhood. Emotions run deep when you're confronted with the prospect of raising a child, mainly because it's a huge commitment and responsibility that, unlike a job, never has time off. Babies are expensive, confusing, time consuming and, for many fathers, represent the end of a carefree 'youth' that has extended well into adulthood.

Experiencing a jumble of feelings is normal, and the more you take those emotions to heart and explore what fatherhood means to you – and what kind of father you want to be – the easier the transition will be when baby arrives.

Looking at the Concept of Fatherhood

What exactly does it mean to be a father? The answer depends on the kind of father you want to be for your child. In recent years, films, TV and even adverts have begun to transition from the bumbling, know-nothing father of yore to the modern dad who is just as comfortable changing a nappy as he is fixing a car. Fathers today range from traditional to equal partners in every aspect of parenting.

The majority of parents nowadays don't adhere to the traditional masculine and feminine roles that our parents and grandparents grew up with. Women work, men work, and caring for the home – inside and out – is both partners' responsibility. Today, fatherhood is a flexible word that's defined by how involved you want to be in the rearing of your child, but the more involved you are in your child's upbringing, the more likely he is to be a well-adjusted, loving and confident person.

A father? Who, me?

Yes, you. As strange as it sounds, you're going to be a father. A great one at that, because just through the mere act of reading this book, you're taking the proverbial bull by the horns and doing your homework to learn what it takes to be a good dad from day one. As they say, anyone can be a father, but it takes someone special to be a dad.

Even if you've never held a baby before, don't let self-doubt rule the day. Being a good father isn't about knowing everything about everything; it's about loving and caring for a baby to the best of your abilities. So don't be afraid. Yes, that's easier said than done, but being fearful of what lies ahead doesn't change the fact that you've got a baby on the way, however far off.

 You may feel silly, but start by saying the words 'I'm going to be a father' out loud a few times. Maybe even look into a mirror while you say it. If the thought of fatherhood scares you, you need to get used to the label, and the more you say and internalise it, the more it will become you.

Reacting to a life-changing event

Dissolving into a tearful, slobbering mess upon finding out that you're going to be a father isn't unusual. Neither is throwing up, passing out, laughing, swearing or any of the normal, healthy reactions people have upon receiving life-altering information.

If your reaction isn't 100 per cent positive, that's okay, too. Just remember that your partner probably won't be particularly thrilled if you get upset, defensive or angry when she tells you she's expecting. As best as you can, react to the news with all the positivity you can muster. You'll have plenty of time to revisit any concerns or frustrations after you've given the situation some time to sink in.

Some dads-to-be go into fix-it mode upon hearing the news, ready and eager to crunch budget numbers, baby-proof the entire home in a single night, begin making university plans 18 years in advance, and so on. Feeling like you need to get everything in order before baby arrives is normal, but remember that you can't do it all in a day, and take some time to celebrate before you dive into the practical side of life with baby. (Turn to Chapter 3 for more on handling the news.)

Dealing with fears of fatherhood

Even men who have been lucky enough to be surrounded by positive male role models for their entire lives still find themselves doubting whether or not they have what it takes to be a dad. This fear resembles that of starting a new job – amplified by 100. Part of being a good father is taking the time to confront your feelings so that when baby comes, you won't be parenting with fear.

Following are some of the common fear-based questions men ask themselves in regard to fatherhood:

- ✔ Am I ready to give up my present life (free time, flexibility, freedom) to be a dad?
- ✔ Will I have time for my pastimes and friends?
- ✔ Will I ever sleep again?
- ✔ Is this the end of my marriage and sex life as I know it?
- ✔ Do we have enough money to raise a child?
- ✔ Do I know enough about kids to be a good dad?
- ✔ Am I mature enough to be a good role model for my child?
- ✔ What if the baby comes and I don't love him?

Your head may be spinning with all of the questions you ask yourself, and although you can't answer them all right away, you need to address them at some point. However, plenty of men have felt unprepared and unwilling and turned out to be great dads, so don't despair if your initial answers to the questions above are mostly negative.

Parenthood involves a lot of sacrifice, but it doesn't have to sound the death knell for your identity or happiness. Talk with your partner, a trusted friend or anyone who will listen to you and support your concerns without getting defensive about the questions you have. Some of your fears, as you'll find, have no basis in reality. Others, such as the fear of losing yourself and your free time, will require you to prioritise your time and energy.

Regardless of what your fears may be, don't let them fester. No man is an island, and you can't effectively deal with all those emotions by yourself. Starting an open dialogue with your partner will keep you both on the same page, which is a good start toward making you an effective parenting duo.

Debunking a few myths about fatherhood

Many of the concerns or fears you likely have originate from the many long-standing myths regarding what a father's role should be in the life of a child. Not all that long ago, men stood in the waiting room at the hospital during delivery and returned to work the next day. The landscape of fatherhood has changed quickly, leaving the modern dad wondering where he fits in the parenting scheme.

Following are some of the most common misconceptions about fatherhood. We debunk those myths to help you understand how to be a more involved father.

Myth number 1: Only the mum-to-be should make decisions about labour and delivery

While the focus is on your partner – she is, after all, the one carrying your child – you also matter, and you have the right to voice your opinions along the way. Throughout the pregnancy, share what you're experiencing and let her know what you're afraid of. She has a lot to think about and worry about, too, but the more you deal with those issues together, the stronger your relationship will become.

If you have thoughts and opinions about what kind of delivery option you're most comfortable with, share those with your partner as well. Although ultimately you need to let her pick the childbirth option that's best for her, she deserves to know your feelings on the matter. Getting involved in the decision-making process isn't just your right; it's the right thing to do. You can turn to Chapter 8 to start finding about the options and many decisions to be made.

Myth number 2: Men aren't ideal caretakers for newborns

Boobs are generally the issue at the forefront of this myth. No, you won't be able to breastfeed your child or know what it's like to give birth. Because they don't have that initial connection, a lot of fathers wonder what exactly they're supposed to do.

Mother and baby are attached to each other for nine months, but after baby arrives, it's open season on bonding and caretaking. When your partner isn't breastfeeding, hold, rock and engage in skin-to-skin contact with your baby. Changing his nappies, bathing and getting him dressed are just a few of the activities that you can do to get involved with your baby. And the more involved you get, the less likely you are to feel left out of the equation. Chapter 10 provides tips for caring for your new baby so you can feel confident in your abilities.

Myth number 3: You will never have sex or sleep ever again

Good things come to those who wait, and you will have to wait. Sex won't happen for at least six weeks following delivery, and even then you have a long road back to being normal. For many couples, a normal sex life following childbirth isn't as active as it once was, but you can work with your partner to make sure both of your needs are being met.

One need that will constrain your sex life – and override the desire for sex – is sleep. Babies don't sleep through the night. They wake up hungry and demand an awake parent to feed them, burp them and soothe them back to sleep. Some babies begin sleeping through the night at six months while other kids won't until the age of three. The good news is that they all sleep through eventually, and when you begin to understand your baby's patterns, you'll be able to figure out a routine that allows you to maximise the shut-eye you get every day.

Myth number 4: Active fathers can't succeed in the business world

Unless work is the only obligation you've ever had in your adult life, you're probably used to juggling more than one thing. Fathers who are active in the community or fill their schedules with copious hours of hobbies will have to re-evaluate their priorities. Family comes first, work comes second, and with the support of a loving partner and a few good babysitters, you'll be able to continue on your career trajectory as planned.

In fact, being a dad may just make you a more effective worker. Having so many demands on your time will make you better at time management and maximising your work day. Focus on work at work and home at home, and you'll succeed in both arenas.

Myth number 5: You're destined to become your father

Destiny is really just a code word for the tendency many men have to mimic the patterns and behaviours that are familiar because they grew up experiencing them. However, if you didn't like an aspect of your father's parenting or don't want to repeat a major mistake that he perpetrated, talk about it with your partner. The more you talk about it, the less likely you are to repeat that mistake because you'll engage your partner as a support system working with you to help you avoid it.

But don't forget to replicate and celebrate the things your father may have done right. You'll be chilled to the bone the first time you say something that your father used to say, but remember that repeating the good actions isn't a bad thing. Don't try to be different from your father 'just because'. Identify what he did that was right and what was wrong, and use that information as a blueprint for your parenting style.

Myth number 6: You'll fall in love with your baby at first sight

Babies aren't always beautiful right after being born, but that's to be expected, given what they've just gone through to enter the world. Don't feel guilty if you look at your baby and aren't immediately enamoured with him. Emotions are difficult to control, and for some fathers – and even mothers – falling head-over-heels for baby may take some time.

Childbirth is a long, intense experience for you as well as your partner (as we describe in Chapter 9), so allow yourself adequate time to rest and get to know the new addition to your family. If you suffer from feelings of regret or extreme sadness, or experience thoughts of harming yourself or the baby, seek immediate medical assistance.

Becoming a Modern Dad

Dads today are involved in every aspect of a child's life. They're no longer relegated to teaching sports, rough-and-tumble and serving as disciplinarians. Modern fatherhood is all about using your strengths, talents and interests to shape your relationship and interactions with your child.

Modern dads change nappies, feed the baby, wake up in the middle of the night to care for a crying child and take baby for a run. They do not 'babysit' their children; they're capable parents, and no job falls outside of the realm of a modern father's capabilities. Though all that involvement does mean you're going to put in far more effort and time than previous generations, it also means that you're bridging the gap of emotional distance that used to be so prevalent in the father–child experience.

In addition to reading the sections below, you can flip to the chapters in Part IV for information and advice on making changes and stepping into the practical role of daddy.

Changes in your personal life

If what you fear most is losing the freedom to spend as much time as you want engaging in leisure activities, then you're in for some mammoth sacrifices. Babies require you to say no to a lot of commitments that the pre-baby you would have agreed to partake in. Don't make a lot of outside-the-home plans that you consider optional, at least at first.

For the first six months, going out at night will be challenging, especially if your partner is breastfeeding, and even more so if you don't live near family. However, as your baby gets older, leaving him with a babysitter becomes more feasible and less stressful.

Perhaps what you fear the most is the impact baby will have on your relationship with your partner. This fear is valid, given that you'll scarcely find time for the two of you to be alone. But that doesn't mean you won't have time to connect.

 Just because going out as a couple is difficult to manage doesn't mean you can't have ample one-to-one time. Plan stay-in dates that start at baby's bedtime. Order food or make a fancy dinner, watch a DVD together or bring out your favourite board game. Try not to talk about baby. Rather, focus on each other and talk about topics that interest you both.

Changes in your professional life

Depending on the requirements of your job, your daily routine may go completely unchanged aside from more yawns in the day resulting from late-night feeds and a nocturnal baby. Thoughts of your new family may make focusing difficult, especially when you first return to work following any paternity leave or holiday you take. In time, you'll settle back into a normal routine, and work just may become the one arena of your life that provides a respite from parenting duties.

Workaholics, however, will find themselves at a crossroads. Some will choose to cut back on hours spent at the office while others, hopefully with the full support of their partners, will proceed with business as usual. No right or wrong way to balance a demanding job with a new baby exists as long as you and your partner are both comfortable with the arrangement and you spend enough quality time with your child.

What is quality time? It's time you spend with your child, focusing *on* your child. Some people say quality time has nothing to do with the quantity of time you spend with your child, but we feel it is affected by the amount of time you devote to your child. Give as much as you can, because the old adage is true – they grow up so fast.

Some dads even leave the workforce altogether or take work-at-home positions in order to provide full-time childcare for their newborn. If you choose this route, make sure to check out Chapter 18, which provides you with an excellent primer for being a successful full-time daddy.

Lifestyle changes to consider

Bad habits are hard to break, but when you have the added stress of a child, those bad habits can be even harder to conquer. That said, you're about to have a child – a sponge who will soak up your every word and action – so it's time to clean up your act.

Following are a few lifestyle alterations to consider making so you can lead by example without reservation:

- **Quit smoking/drinking too much/taking recreational drugs.** Second-hand smoke increases the risk of illness for your child, as well as the likelihood that he'll become a smoker as an adult. Frequent overconsumption of alcohol makes you less likely to be a responsible parent capable of making good, safe decisions for your baby. In fact, alcohol and drugs often lead to harmful and neglectful decisions that can land you in legal trouble and your child in the foster care system.

- **Start an exercise regimen.** Physically active, healthy parents get less run down and are less susceptible to illness. Plus, you'll want to live a long life with your children.

- ✔ **Lose weight.** If you're heavily overweight, you're more susceptible to illness and a shortened life span, and furthermore, children of obese parents are more likely to be obese. Kids learn nutrition and lifestyle habits from their parents, so set a good example and give your child a fair shot at a long and healthy life.

- ✔ **Eat more healthily.** Your partner needs to be extremely diligent about eating pregnancy-positive foods, so use this time as an opportunity to get your diet in order. Soon enough, you'll be cooking for three, and if you're already in the habit of preparing healthy foods, you'll have no trouble providing proper nutrition for your child.

- ✔ **Control your anger/censor your bad language.** Children learn how to treat and interact with others at a very young age. Start revising your behaviour now and get used to swearing less, before your kid picks up some nasty communication habits.

- ✔ **Spend less money on non-essential items.** Teaching kids fiscal responsibility is just as important as teaching them social responsibility. Plus, kids aren't cheap, so it'd be an idea to stop spending £30 a week on beer and start banking your savings to provide a sound, secure future for your family.

- ✔ **Organise and de-clutter your home.** Create a safe, livable place for your new addition, and in doing so also help decrease the amount of stress in your life.

- ✔ **Develop routines.** Be it running errands, cooking, making or receiving phone calls or paying the bills, get systems in place to ensure that everything gets done with the least amount of hair pulling. Knowing who does what when keeps you on track when baby throws a wrench into everything.

Deciding to Take the Plunge (Or Not)

For some of you, the question of whether or not you're ready for fatherhood comes too late. Others may be reading this book as a first step in planning for the future. Deciding on the right time in life to have a baby isn't an easy task, especially because circumstances change on a seemingly daily basis.

However, family planning is an essential step that can minimise what ifs, frustrations and regrets. Once you have a baby, you can't take it back. Knowing when you're ready to be parents and then trying to conceive means that when you actually do get pregnant, the time will indeed be right.

Determining whether you're ready

How does it feel when you know you want to be a father? And how can you know when you're actually ready to start trying for a baby? Those questions have no simple answers, because the feeling is different for everyone, but suffice it to say, you'll know when you know.

One sign to look for is a prolonged interest in and fascination with the babies of friends and family members. Women call the growing desire for a baby a *biological clock*, and many men experience similar feelings. The desire to procreate, to have your genes carried on in the species, can be powerful.

Just make sure it's a desire that lasts more than a day. Also, make sure that you take the time to analyse the impact a baby is going to have on your life. If you're in the final two years of a college course, it may be in your best interest to wait. If you're unemployed, perhaps you want to put off trying until you find a job you like that can support a family.

Just because you're ready doesn't make now the right time. Don't decide to have a baby on an impulse. Think about the impact a child will have on your time, money and home, and if you don't see any major obstacles, then by all means, proceed. Obviously you can choose to proceed even if having a baby now doesn't make sense on every level, but please make sure first that you can provide a loving, safe home and can pay for all the things a baby needs to thrive.

Telling your partner you're ready

You can tell your partner anytime and anyplace that you're ready to take the plunge into parenthood, but however you broach the subject, remember that she may not be as ready as you. A good way to introduce the subject is by asking her questions about her feelings on when the right time is to have a baby.

Tell her how excited you are, but also let her know that you've thought about the finances and logistics of having a baby, too. Fatherhood involves a lot more than choosing a name and a nursery theme. A big part of feeling ready is knowing that the person you're going to have a baby with isn't just enamoured with the idea of a baby but is also prepared for the practicalities of responsibly starting a family.

You don't have to outline every aspect of how and why you're ready, but treat the idea with respect and let your partner know you're sincere by proving that you've actually thought it through.

Telling your partner you're not ready

If your partner is already pregnant, do not under any circumstances tell her you're not ready. If, however, the two of you simply are exploring the idea of having a child, now is the perfect time to speak your piece and let her know that you're just not prepared for fatherhood.

Reasons for not being ready vary from practical (not enough money or time) to logistical (still at college, caring for a sick parent) to selfish (not ready to share the Xbox). No reason to not be ready is wrong, but if your partner is ready for a baby, don't expect her to be fully supportive.

Regardless, don't agree to have a child before you're up for the challenge just so that your partner doesn't get angry with you. Be honest, because when she's pregnant, you can't do anything to change the situation. If you're uncertain now, be honest and speak up!

Being patient when one of you is ready (and the other isn't)

Being on different pages can be an uncomfortable position for any couple, especially when it comes to the child issue. Men have long been saddled with the Peter Pan label whenever they announce they aren't ready to 'grow up' and have kids. Women are unfairly chastised for choosing career over family if they aren't ready to have a child.

Everyone has reasons for wanting or not wanting to have a baby, and every one of them is valid – at least to the person who isn't ready. Attempting to persuade your partner, or vice versa, to have a baby is not recommended. Having a child with someone who isn't ready is setting up your relationship – and your relationship with the child – for failure.

If one of you isn't ready, try to work out a timeline as to when the wary party will be ready. If you can't set a definitive date, choose a time when you will revisit the topic. Check in with each other on the topic at least every six months. Nagging the other person isn't a good idea, but if it's something one of you wants, then you should continue to work toward a solution.

Seek counselling at any point if you and your partner are fighting about the issue frequently, or if one of you makes the decision that you never want children. Couples who find themselves at an impasse about whether or not they will have children often need the guidance of a trained professional.

Dealing with an unexpected pregnancy

Unplanned pregnancies aren't uncommon, and, for the majority of people in a committed relationship, adjusting to the surprising news is often no more than a minor bump in the road. If you unexpectedly find out that you're going to be a dad, don't get angry with your partner. Blaming the other person is easy when emotions run high, but don't forget how you got into this situation in the first place. It does, indeed, take two.

Birth control and family planning are the responsibility of both the man and the woman, and accidents sometimes happen. The best thing you can do in this instance is to talk with your partner about your options and start making a plan about how to give that child the best life you possibly can. Having a child unexpectedly isn't the end of the world, and you don't have to feel ready to have a baby to be a good father.

Welcoming long-awaited pregnancies

Getting pregnant isn't always as easy as they make it look in films, as the millions of infertile couples know all too well. (And if you and your partner are dealing with infertility, turn to Chapter 2 for help.) Finding out that you're pregnant after a long wait brings a mixed bag of emotions, most of which are joyful.

If you and your partner have been struggling to get pregnant, you likely feel relieved that you're about to get the gift you've been working so hard for, but don't be surprised if you have difficulty adjusting to life outside of the infertility world. After months and years of scheduled sex, countless hospital visits and suffering month after month of disappointment, not everyone transitions into the pregnancy phase with ease.

You also may struggle with a sense of fear resulting from previous miscarriages, close calls and years of disappointment. Make sure to allow yourselves the opportunity to gripe, complain, worry and grieve for a process that took a lot of patience and energy. Frustrations that were bottled up for the sake of optimism may finally surface, which is absolutely healthy.

Just because you've finally achieved your goal doesn't make all the feelings of sadness and frustration suddenly disappear. If you and/ or your partner are having trouble letting go of the feelings that gripped you during your fertility struggle, you can find countless support groups, online communities and blogs that provide both of you with a place to talk about what you've been through. You can also learn transition tips from others who have been through the same thing. Moving forward will get easier, but it can take time – and sometimes a lot of support.

Glimpsing into the Pregnancy Process Ahead

When you get used to the idea of being a father (which you hope- fully will), you may wonder what comes next. For the uninitiated, first-time dad, the nine months of pregnancy are a whirlwind of planning, worrying, parties, nesting, name searching, doctor visits and information gathering as you move toward baby's birth. In the following sections we lay out what you can expect in each *trimester* (a period of three months).

First trimester

In the first trimester, which encompasses the first three months of pregnancy, your partner suffers from the majority of pregnancy symptoms, such as nausea, intense sleepiness, unexplained tears and the all-important cravings.

By the end of the first trimester, your baby is about 3 or 4 inches (7.5–10cm) in length and weighs approximately 1 ounce (28g). At that time, your baby's arms, legs, hands and feet are fully formed, and he's able to open and close his fists. The circulatory and uri- nary systems are fully functional. Secondary body parts, such as fingernails, teeth and reproductive organs, begin developing. Turn to Chapter 3 for more information on what happens during the first trimester.

Second trimester

During the second trimester, most of your partner's early preg- nancy symptoms disappear, but her body undergoes visible changes. She begins to look and feel pregnant, and may begin struggling with the not-so-fun aspects of carrying a child, such as weight gain and forgetfulness.

This is also the time when the fun stuff begins. Around week 20, your partner has the ultrasound that can determine the sex of the baby – if you choose to find out and if the baby allows the ultra-sound technician a clear view. It's also the time when you prepare the nursery, weed through countless baby names, attend antenatal classes and baby-proof your house.

By the end of the second trimester, your baby is roughly 14inches (35.5cm) long and weighs approximately 2 pounds (0.9kg). His skin is still translucent, but his eyes begin to open and close, and your partner is likely to start feeling movements and even baby's tiny hiccups. Check out Chapter 4 to find out more about the second trimester.

Third trimester

Assuming all goes according to plan and your baby goes full-term (that is, he isn't premature) or somewhere close to it, the third tri-mester is one of the longest three-month periods of your life. Your partner begins to feel uncomfortable as the size of her body makes it difficult to move and sleep in a normal way, and you both get anxious about the impending arrival.

To make the most of the time, you and your partner need to take care of business, such as picking a hospital you're comfortable, crafting your birth plan, getting your maternity and paternity leave sorted out, creating a phone tree to announce baby's arrival and finishing up any odd projects around the house that need to be done before the big day.

During the third trimester, your baby is fully developed and focused on growing larger and stronger for life on the outside. This is also the last time for many, many years that you and your part-ner exist solely as a couple, so be sure to take the time to indulge yourselves in the things you love to do together. Life may feel like it's on pause for at least the first six months of baby's existence, so get out now and enjoy the freedom of childlessness. Soon enough, your life will be a lot more complicated and busy – and happy, too. Very, very happy. Chapter 7 gives you more information on what to expect and do in the third trimester.

While You Were Gestating

Because the first few weeks of pregnancy will probably be rather uneventful, now is a good time to start a time capsule for the year your baby will be born. Many years down the road, when your child is an adult, it will be a touching, informative look back at the time when he entered the world. For you and your partner, it will be a fun, celebratory action to kick off the pregnancy festivities.

Keep cinema tickets, take-out menus, a newspaper from the day you found out your partner was pregnant (as well as clippings of the most important headlines of the year), favourite ads, magazine clippings, and so on. Make a mix CD of the most popular songs, as well as one of your favourite music.

As you choose names, add the list of all potential names into the time capsule. When you choose a paint colour for the nursery, put in the paint colour card. Any decision you and your partner make for the baby is a good candidate for inclusion. It may seem silly now, but in 20 years it will be the best gift you can give your child.

Chapter 2

Beyond the Bed: Conception Basics

*Y*ou may have spent years trying not to get pregnant, so the change from not trying to trying can be mind-boggling. Something even the most clueless people manage to do effortlessly can cause you to lose sleep at night and turn sex into a job. Getting pregnant is hard work sometimes.

In this chapter we cover how to make the getting pregnant process not just painless, but fun, even if it takes longer than you expected.

Understanding Conception

You can't get pregnant any old time you want; your partner has to be ovulating and releasing an egg, and you have to be sending some good swimmers her way. The whole baby-making process can be so complex that it seems like a miracle people are on earth at all. This section tells you about the mechanics of how eggs and sperm actually get together and what they need from the two of you.

Baby-making basics

Getting pregnant requires that several players be on the scene at the right time: namely, good sperm and a mature egg. If the two meet in the fallopian tube, which is the conduit from the ovary down to the uterus, join together to form a fertilised egg and then float down to a uterus with a lining that's exactly the right thickness to facilitate implantation, pregnancy occurs. If any of those factors are amiss, well, that's when things get complicated.

Producing a mature egg

Before she's even born, a woman has all the eggs she'll ever have. Unlike sperm, no new eggs are being produced; the original eggs are just matured, usually one at a time. Mature eggs are produced from immature ones (called oocytes), located in the ovaries, through a complex interaction of three hormones during the menstrual cycle. Those hormones – oestradiol (a form of oestrogen), follicle stimulating hormone (FSH) and luteinising hormone (LH) – work like this:

1. FSH stimulates the ovaries, which produce oestrogen.

2. Oestradiol production starts to mature a number of egg-containing follicles, small cyst-like structures that contain the immature eggs.

3. One follicle, called a lead follicle, continues to develop while the rest atrophy.

4. Around day 14 of the menstrual cycle, LH kicks in to mature the egg and move it to the centre of the follicle so it can release.

5. The egg releases from the follicle and begins to float down the fallopian tube. This is where you come in.

Figure 2-1 shows the events of a menstrual cycle when pregnancy does not occur.

Sending in some good sperm

Sperm can only fertilise an egg that's mature, so you need to either have sperm waiting in the fallopian tube when the egg is released or get some there within 12 to 24 hours after ovulation, because that's how long the egg can live. Sperm (shown in Figure 2-2) live for at least a few days, so having sex the day before ovulation, or even two days before, is usually adequate. If your partner is monitoring her ovulation, give it one more shot the day of ovulation.

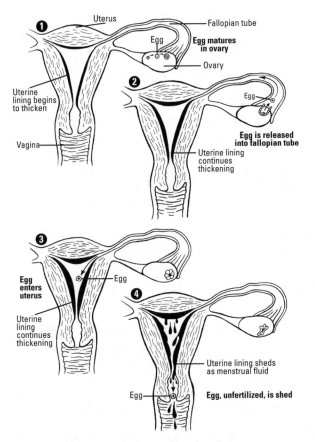

Figure 2-1: Every event in the menstrual cycle has a purpose.

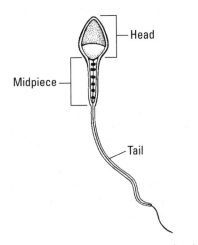

Figure 2-2: Sperm are compact swimming machines.

Why so many sperm?

Women produce one egg a month, most of the time, and men produce millions of sperm. You may wonder, why the huge disparity? Because of the inability of one sperm to do the honours. Only one sperm makes it into the egg, but it takes many sperm to break down the coating that surrounds the egg. And while eggs get to drift downward from the ovary to the fallopian tube, sperm have to swim upstream. Needless to say, some fall by the wayside.

Sperm also are produced in large quantities because many are abnormal, having two tails, no tails, round tails, small heads, large heads or abnormally shaped heads. Abnormal tails make navigation difficult, and abnormal heads often indicate chromosomal abnormalities.

Only 50 to 60 per cent of sperm need good motility, or movement, for a sperm sample to be considered normal, so lots of sperm don't make the grade, creating a need for a high quantity.

Making the journey and attaching to the uterus

After fertilisation, the new potential life has to make it down the tube to the uterus, where it implants. The journey from the fallopian tube to uterus takes between five to seven days, on average, and implantation normally occurs seven to ten days after conception. The fallopian tube is normally a fairly straight tube, but if it's been damaged by infection so that it's twisted or dilated, the embryo may wander around in the folds and never get to the uterus.

Even worse, the embryo may implant in the tube, which is an *ectopic pregnancy*. The tube has no room for a developing foetus, so an ectopic pregnancy is doomed from the start and can cause serious, life-threatening bleeding if the tube ruptures.

Even after the embryo reaches the uterus, implantation isn't always plain sailing. The uterine lining has to be just right for implantation. Oestrogen thickens the lining before ovulation, and progesterone released from the corpus luteum, the leftover shell of the follicle that contained the egg, prepares the lining after ovulation.

After the embryo reaches the uterus and implants, the implanting embryo begins to produce human chorionic gonadotropin, or hCG, the hormone that pregnancy tests measure. hCG levels aren't detectable until the embryo implants, or around the time of the first missed period.

Conception statistics

If you don't get pregnant in the first month you try, you may immediately start worrying. But bear in mind that pregnancy is by no means a sure thing, even when you do everything right and have no major fertility issues. According to statistics:

- ✔ Out of 100 couples under age 35 trying to get pregnant in a given month, 20 will achieve their goal, but three will miscarry.

- ✔ If your partner is in her late thirties, you have a 10 per cent chance of pregnancy each month, but a 34 per cent chance of miscarriage.

- ✔ If she's older than 40, you have only a 5 per cent chance of pregnancy each month, and more than a 50 per cent chance of miscarriage.

The good news is that 75 out of 100 30-year-olds trying to get pregnant will become pregnant within a year of trying, and 66 per cent of 35-year-olds will get pregnant in a year. Around 44 per cent of 40-year-olds become pregnant within a year. Over age 40, variables such as hormone levels affect pregnancy rates, and generalisations are hard to make.

Answering commonly asked questions about getting pregnant

Getting pregnant may seem straightforward, but what exactly does it take? Here are some answers to the most common concerns:

- ✔ **How long does it take?**

  On average, more than half of couples get pregnant within the first six months of trying and four out of five are pregnant within one year.

- ✔ **Does having more sex increase the chances of pregnancy?**

  No. In fact, due to the amount of time it takes for semen volume to build back up to normal levels following ejaculation, overdoing it around ovulation time by having sex several times a day can deplete your sperm count, which probably won't be a problem if you have a normal sperm count, but can be if your count is low.

✔ **Should we only have sex with my partner on her back and me on top?**

It's a myth that this standard position is the best way to get pregnant. While it may help the semen stay in better, no scientific proof exists that the sexual position you choose has any effect on conception rates.

✔ **Does my partner's past use of the birth control pill mean it will take longer?**

It varies from person to person. One woman can miss a single pill and end up pregnant while others may take a little longer. Just remember, the chances of getting pregnant in the first month are small, but the average couple is pregnant within a year regardless of past birth-control usage.

✔ **Is it okay to drink and smoke when trying to conceive?**

If you're ready to be pregnant, you should give up smoking immediately. Having an occasional drink or two when you're trying to become a mum or dad is unlikely to produce a negative outcome, but the general rule of thumb is to live as though your partner is pregnant from the moment you begin trying to conceive. Check out the next section for more tips on getting healthy to improve the odds of conception.

Evaluating Health to Get Ready for Parenthood

Some health issues and bad habits can make it harder to get pregnant. A few months before trying to get pregnant, take an inventory of behaviours and health issues and get yourselves into the best shape possible, not only so that you can get pregnant without difficulty but also so you'll be healthy new parents.

Checking out your physical health before trying to get pregnant isn't difficult. See your doctor, let her know you're trying to get pregnant, change any medications that may impact fertility and take some blood tests.

Uncovering female health issues that impact conception

Many female health problems can cause fertility difficulties. Some affect egg production and the menstrual cycle; others affect egg transport and implantation, like fibroids and fallopian tube damage. Many can be improved after you identify them.

Sexually transmitted diseases

One of the biggest fertility busters in the age of sexual freedom is sexually transmitted diseases, or STDs. The following STDs can affect female fertility in these ways:

- ✔ Chlamydia, if not treated promptly, increases by 40 per cent the risk of pelvic inflammatory disease (PID), which damages the fallopian tubes. Women with PID are seven to ten times more likely to have an ectopic pregnancy. Eighty per cent of women who have had chlamydia three or more times are infertile.

- ✔ Gonorrhoea also increases the risk of PID and ectopic pregnancy.

- ✔ Syphilis can cause miscarriage, stillbirth, and developmental delays and blindness in your unborn child.

STDs need to be treated early with antibiotics before damage is done to the fallopian tubes.

Endometriosis

Endometriosis, implantation of the tissue that lines the inside of the uterus in places it doesn't belong, is common; 2 million women in the UK suffer from it, and 40 per cent of women with endometriosis have fertility issues.

Endometriosis tissue bleeds at the time of the menstrual period and leads to scarring and pain. Endometrial implants can be removed in some cases, but they tend to recur. Most endometriosis is found in the pelvis, near the uterus, but it can turn up in some odd places, like the lungs. In vitro fertilisation (IVF) can increase the chances of pregnancy in women with endometriosis.

Polycystic ovary syndrome

Polycystic ovary syndrome, PCOS, affects between 5 to 10 per cent of women of childbearing age, and can cause *anovulation*, or failure to produce a mature egg. PCOS is associated with an abnormal rise in male hormones, called androgens; all women have some male hormones, but women with PCOS have more than normal. They're often overweight and have excess body and facial hair, thinning head hair (just like some men) and acne. Women with PCOS also have higher rates of type 2 diabetes, heart disease, high cholesterol and high blood pressure. Fertility medications may be needed for women with PCOS to get pregnant.

Thyroid problems

Thyroid problems are common in women of childbearing age and can cause anovulation (failure to recruit and develop eggs). A simple blood test checks for thyroid function. Low thyroid levels can raise prolactin levels, which can also interfere with ovulation.

Fibroids

Fibroids are common uterine growths (rarely cancerous) that occur in up to 75 per cent of women and often cause no problems with conception. However, fibroids can grow big enough to interfere with embryo implantation or cause premature labour in some women. See Figure 2-3.

Fibroids are easily seen with pelvic ultrasound, and can be removed surgically if they appear to be interfering with pregnancy.

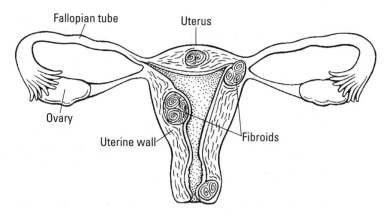

Figure 2-3: Fibroids grow into the uterine lining and occasionally interfere with pregnancy.

Recognising issues that cause fertility problems in men

Sperm take a long time to make. Sperm you ejaculate today have been three months in the making, so if you're working on health problems or making lifestyle changes, give them enough time to take effect.

While male health issues may seem less important to a quick conception, your health problems can interfere with conception. Here are a few examples of potentially problematic issues:

✔ Diabetic men often have problems with erection and ejaculation. Presumably if you have a problem with erection, you're
already well aware of it, but ejaculatory issues may not be
quite as obvious. Retrograde ejaculation, where sperm get
pushed into the bladder rather than out through the urethra,
can affect diabetic men.

✔ Men who take high-blood-pressure medications called calcium
channel blockers may have sperm that don't penetrate eggs
well; other blood pressure medications may cause retrograde
ejaculation.

✔ Toxins common to the workplace, such as lead, X-rays or
inhaled anaesthetics in the operating theatre, and a host of
other environmentally damaging substances can also be
damaging your internal plumbing if you work with them
frequently.

✔ STDs can also take their toll on the male reproductive system.
Chlamydia and gonorrhoea can cause an infection and inflammation in the epididymis, part of the testes where sperm
develop. Syphilis can cause low sperm count and poor motility.

Assessing lifestyle choices that affect eggs and sperm

You can impact your chances of pregnancy every month with your
lifestyle choices. Yes, giving up bad habits is painful, but not getting pregnant month after month is pretty painful, too. Take the
step of cutting the following bad habits out of your life before you
start trying to get pregnant.

Smoking

Smoking can affect sperm and eggs and increase miscarriage
rates. In the UK, nearly one in five adults smoke. If either of you is
a smoker, quit for at least a few months before trying to get pregnant. Quitting may help you avoid these pitfalls:

✔ Smokers have sperm that are less motile (capable of moving
spontaneously). They have a long way to go to reach the egg,
so they need all the motility they can get.

✔ Smokers have lower sperm counts and more abnormally
shaped sperm, which are chromosomally abnormal.

✔ Female smokers have more eggs that are chromosomally
abnormal.

✔ Female smokers have a 50 per cent higher chance of miscarriage.

✔ Female smokers are two to four times more likely to have an ectopic pregnancy (a pregnancy that implants outside the uterus).

Drinking alcohol

Alcohol has far-reaching issues for the foetus long past the moment of conception, so cutting out alcohol before trying to get pregnant and avoiding it like the plague after getting pregnant are essential for your partner. It won't hurt you, either. Heavy drinking, three or more drinks a day for a guy, can decrease sperm quantity and quality. And a drink doesn't have to be hard spirits; one beer is a drink.

Using drugs

Two commonly used drugs can affect male fertility: marijuana and anabolic steroids. Marijuana lowers testosterone levels in males, and testosterone is the male hormone responsible for male sexual functioning and sperm production. Sperm counts are lower and sperm is less motile in men who use marijuana regularly.

Steroid use is more common than you may think: around 4 to 5 per cent of all men in the UK have used steroids to build muscle mass. Steroids suppress testosterone production and can cause irreversible damage to the sperm production line. Avoid anabolic steroids at all costs.

Maintaining a healthy weight

Unfortunately, being overweight is a huge problem, and it's getting bigger all the time. Around half of women of childbearing age in the UK are overweight or obese. Women who are overweight may not ovulate, and if they don't ovulate, they can't get pregnant. One Australian study showed that obese women were only half as likely to get pregnant as normal-weight women.

However, being underweight can also interfere with ovulation. Overall, 12 per cent of infertility issues are related to being over- or underweight. Fortunately, either losing or gaining weight in these cases results in pregnancy 70 per cent of the time.

Issues that may never have crossed your mind

Sometimes behaviours you may never have considered can negatively impact your partner's chances of pregnancy. Here are a few:

✔ **Douching:** Although between one-third to one-half of women of childbearing age do it, *douching* (rinsing out the vagina with water or chemicals) is not only unnecessary, it's potentially harmful. Women who douche are 73 per cent more likely to have pelvic inflammatory disease, which can seriously damage the fallopian tubes and increases the chance of ectopic pregnancy by about the same percentage.

And because you want your partner around for a long time, remind her of this statistic: women who douche are 80 per cent more likely to develop cervical cancer.

✔ **Not sitting on the couch enough:** No, not really – some exercise is definitely good for you. But some sports, like bicycling, may cause testicular damage from the pressure of the bike seat. Women who exercise too heavily may stop having periods (called *amenorrhea*), and good luck getting pregnant without them.

✔ **Spending time in hot tubs and other heat sources:** Hot tubs, tight underwear, saunas, steam rooms and anything else that raises the temperature of the testicles is bad for the boys. Hot tubs may also damage eggs and increase miscarriage rates, so neither of you should be lolling in one.

Keeping Sex from Becoming a Chore

As unfathomable as it seems, sex while trying to conceive isn't always fun. Couples often begin to feel a sense of duty and pressure when they move from spontaneity to planning exactly when to have sex to increase their chances of conception. Monitoring rises in body temperature, charting mucus and even lying down afterward to give the semen time to do its job are just a few of the unromantic actions that can take your sex life from crackin' to clinical.

Pleasure may seem to take a back seat to the goal of having a baby, and nothing takes the 'sexy' out of sex faster than making it feel like work. In fact, if the sex becomes solely about trying to conceive, you may begin to feel a bit like a sperm-producing machine that's only needed during ovulation, and performance issues can arise (no pun intended).

If for some reason conception takes a while, this feeling will only increase as you both grow impatient. If you begin to suffer these feelings, share them with your partner immediately. Plan 'sex dates' that don't revolve around conception time, and discuss ways to create a more relaxing, less stressful, romantic environment.

Choosing the best time for conception

We're not talking about the phase of the moon or the alignment of the stars here; we're talking about planning to have sex at certain times to increase the odds that you'll hit the day when an egg is present and ready to be fertilised. Not all women have 28-day menstrual cycles, and ovulation doesn't always occur on day 14 of the cycle. Ovulation does always occur 12 to 14 days before the next period is due, or, to be more accurate, your partner's period starts 12 to 14 days after ovulation occurs. You can figure out the best timing for your conception efforts in several ways, which we explore in the following sections.

Monitoring ovulation with a kit

Predicting ovulation doesn't take mind-reading abilities. Simple observation and a few ovulation predictor kits from the chemist are all you need to pinpoint the big day. Ovulation predictor kits (OPKs) pinpoint the rise in luteinising hormone that occurs just before egg release. Your partner urinates into a cup, and then dips the test stick into the urine and reads the results.

The only drawback to OPKs is that women who have high levels of LH (luteinising hormone – what a pregnancy test detects) normally [sense of 'normally' here?], like women in or near menopause and women with PCOS, may not get accurate results.

Watching for physical signs of ovulation

Your partner may also be able to tell when ovulation occurs by these signs:

- ✔ Cervical mucus becomes more copious, thinner, and more slippery and stretchy as ovulation approaches.

- ✔ She may have *mittelschmerz*, a pain on the left or right side as the egg releases from the ovary.

- ✔ Her temperature drops slightly right before ovulation and rises afterward.

Ovulation can be tracked by keeping a monthly temperature chart, but it can be a real pain because she has to take her temperature first thing in the morning, before she gets out of bed, uses the bathroom or has a cup of coffee.

Catching ovulation with a regular visit

If you don't want to closely monitor ovulation, you can take the easy way and simply have sex on a frequent, regular schedule. Doctors seem to have differing opinions on how much sex is enough when you're trying to get pregnant. Some say every other day helps build up a good supply of sperm; some say every day is okay, starting a few days before ovulation and continuing (if you're not exhausted!) until the day after ovulation.

The most sensible schedule suggests having sex every other day, all month if you're up for it, starting right after her period ends. Since sperm live for up to five days, having sex the day before ovulation or the day of ovulation gives you a good shot at fertilisation, and if you're aiming for every other day, you're bound to hit one or the other.

Looking at do's and don'ts for scheduling sex

Just because you've written sex down on your calendar doesn't mean it's just another obligation that eats up your time and lacks excitement. After all, this appointment has a far bigger upside than the average visit to the dentist.

Since you have only a few ideal times each month to conceive, you need to make time for sex on those days, which requires planning ahead. Follow these do's and don'ts to make sure your sex life doesn't suffer for the sake of conception.

Do:

- ✔ **Put it on your calendar.** While the planning may seem unsexy, it can be very exciting to look forward to intercourse all week. In fact, verbal foreplay leading up to intercourse will only increase the excitement.

- ✔ **Plan a date that night if possible to make it a fully-fledged romantic evening.** Making it just about the sex will increase the pressure to perform.

- ✔ **Engage in foreplay.** On TV and in films, you often see the ovulating woman demand sex the minute her body temperature leads her to believe it's the best time. Make sure to keep it romantic and intimate. Some light massage, touching and kissing should do the trick.

✔ **Mix it up.** Remember that though some positions are supposed to be better when trying to conceive [earlier the text said there was no evidence that certain positions improved chances of conception], that doesn't mean you have to stay in the same one the whole time.

✔ **Keep it spontaneous.** Knowing the exact date you're going to have sex doesn't mean the setting has to stay the same. Play music, light candles, take a warm bath (not too hot – remember, you don't want to overheat the boys!), or even play out a fantasy if your partner is game.

✔ **Help make the aftermath enjoyable.** Your partner may want to elevate her legs and stay in bed for a while after intercourse to give the semen the best chance to stay put. Help her elevate her legs, and then put on her favourite show or read to her from a book. Don't just get up and leave her alone.

✔ **Have unscheduled sex.** Letting nature run its course every once in a while is okay, even when your road to conception is more like driving in bumper-to-bumper traffic than cruising along on the motorway. After ejaculation, sperm can live in a woman's reproductive tract for up to five days.

Don't:

✔ **Try too hard.** Sex carries its own set of complex, anxiety-inducing expectations, but now that the expectations include creating a baby, the pressure can become downright overwhelming. If you experience performance issues, either mental or physical, due to the stress of the moment, talk about it with your partner. You won't do anyone a favour by having sex as if you're taking a driving test.

✔ **Talk about the baby.** Unless talking about getting her pregnant is a turn-on to your partner, keep the baby discussion out of the sex equation. Although trying to have a baby does indeed require sex, talking about getting her pregnant while engaging in intercourse likely won't set your bedroom on fire.

✔ **Drink before you have sex.** Alcohol can cause performance issues, and the last thing you want to do is let your partner down because you had one too many beers.

✔ **Assume your partner isn't interested in both pleasure and conception.** In fact, studies show that women who orgasm have a greater chance of conceiving than those who don't.

Taking a Brief Yet Important Look at Infertility

Around one in six or seven couples in the UK may have difficulty conceiving (approximately 3.5 million people.) However, the number of couples who are actually infertile is low, around 5 per cent.

Couples under the age of 35 are diagnosed with infertility following 12 months of attempted reproduction that do not yield a pregnancy.

Knowing the facts about infertility

Imagine 100 average couples under the age of 35 trying to get pregnant – the following outcomes are expected:

- ✔ 75 couples are pregnant within a year.

- ✔ 10 couples are pregnant after two years of trying without medical intervention.

- ✔ 10 couples need treatment from an infertility specialist in order to conceive.

Causes of infertility can be complex and often hard to diagnose. Some are related to health and lifestyle issues discussed in the 'Evaluating Health to Get Ready for Parenthood' section earlier in this chapter. Despite treatments and diagnostic practices that primarily focus on women, the statistics paint a different picture:

- ✔ One-third of infertility is diagnosed as female-factor.

- ✔ One-third of infertility is diagnosed as male-factor.

- ✔ Between 10 and 15 per cent of infertility cases are diagnosed as a combination of male- and female-factor.

- ✔ About 20 per cent of infertility cases are unexplained following diagnostic testing.

For women, the main causes of infertility are

- ✔ **Ovulatory disorders:** No ovulation or ovulation on an irregular schedule.

- ✔ **Tubal disorders:** Fallopian tubes are blocked or have an infection that interferes with ovulation or sperm travel.

- ✔ **Uterine issues:** Fibroids (non-cancerous tumours in the uterus) and polyps (growths that can cause blockages).

For men, the main causes of infertility are

✔ **Low sperm count:** Not enough guys to get the job done.

✔ **Decreased sperm motility:** The sperm has trouble moving forward into the fallopian tubes.

✔ **Abnormally shaped sperm:** Abnormal shapes usually indicate chromosomal abnormalities.

✔ **No sperm present in the ejaculate:** A blockage somewhere in the reproductive tract or hormonal disorders can cause an absence of sperm.

Checking on potential problems when nothing's happening

For many couples, the first step toward fixing infertility is admitting that you're having a problem. This revelation isn't easy to make, because it means that at some basic level your bodies are failing you. Fertility problems aren't fair, they're not fun and they can cause a wide array of emotions and frustrations and even outright anger.

The good news is that we live in an age in which getting pregnant doesn't have to be a simple matter of the birds and the bees. Throw in a doctor or two, and you may be well on your way to conceiving in no time flat.

If you're not getting pregnant after a few months, especially if your partner is older than 35, it's time to check things out – for both of you. For her, this may involve the following tests:

✔ **Blood tests:** These check hormone levels, including follicle stimulating hormone, or FSH. FSH levels are normally below 9 mIU/ml on day two or three of the menstrual cycle; higher levels indicate decreased ovarian reserve and the possible need for medical intervention.

✔ **Hysterosalpingogram (HSG):** This test injects dye into the uterus through a catheter placed through the cervix. The dye outlines the shape of the uterus and fallopian tubes. HSG can identify blockages in or dilation of the fallopian tubes that interferes with embryo transport, and it also shows fibroids and polyps in the uterus, which may interfere with implantation.

> ✔ **Pelvic ultrasound scan and hysteroscopy:** If a pelvic ultrasound scan indicates the presence of fibroids or polyps (small growths that can interfere with implantation), a hysteroscopy may be needed. This test uses an endoscope, a sort of mini-telescope, to evaluate the uterus for fibroids or polyps. Small fibroids and polyps can also be removed at the time of the test.

For you, it's a trip to the GP for a physical examination, some simple blood tests and a semen analysis. A semen analysis is the only way you can discover your sperm count and the quality and motility of your sperm.

Collection of semen is just as uncomfortable as it sounds, but it must be done. Just keep your expectations to a minimum and forget those film scenes showing posh rooms, dirty magazines and absolute privacy. If you have to produce in a hospital lab, you may very well find yourself in a toilet, unable to escape the distractions of screaming children and the chatter of nursing staff outside your cubicle.

Some hospitals allow specimens to be collected in the privacy of your home and then delivered to the lab within an hour. Ask your doctor about this alternative, as well as any special instructions for collection and transportation.

Working through it when your partner needs treatment

Some female fertility issues are easily dealt with by simply taking a pill that induces ovulation. But female infertility can also lead to daily injections of fertility medications, uncomfortable vaginal ultrasounds to assess egg development, painful surgeries to remove fibroids or repair damaged fallopian tubes and frequent blood tests.

Fixing female fertility issues can be a drawn-out affair that combines inconvenient and uncomfortable procedures with medications that manipulate hormones, a difficult combination if there ever was one. And if she suddenly views childbearing as a woman's most important prerogative, her seeming inability to accomplish it and subsequent emotions can make fertility treatment a tough time for both of you.

Even though you may have your own stresses when dealing with fertility issues, remember that at least you aren't dealing with a barrage of excess hormones, and keep your cool if conversations get complicated.

Exploring solutions when your sperm don't stack up

A count of less than 20 million is considered a low sperm count. Although that may sound like a large number, because of the number of abnormal sperm in the normal sample as well as the distance required to reach the egg, it takes a lot of good sperm to achieve conception.

Sperm is produced in a cycle, so the semen you produce now actually was created three months ago. If your sperm count is low, start by thinking back to what was going on then. An illness, medication or a weekend in a hot tub may be the culprit.

Understanding the components

What exactly makes a semen specimen normal? The following guidelines from the World Health Organization (WHO) are deemed the ideal for baby-making:

- ✔ **Volume:** About 1.5 to 5 millilitres of semen should be present in a single ejaculate, equalling about a teaspoon.

- ✔ **Concentration:** Strength in numbers is key. You'll need at least 20 million sperm per millilitre of ejaculate to hit the normal range.

- ✔ **Motility:** For every man, an average ejaculate contains dead, slow and immobile sperm. However, at least 40 per cent of your sperm in a single sample should be moving.

- ✔ **Morphology:** Shape is also important to reproduction, and the lab technician examining your sample takes a close look at how many of your swimmers are normally shaped. A normal amount of normally shaped sperm is considered to be anything above 30 per cent.

- ✔ **Trajectory:** Graded on a four-point scale, this test determines how many of your sperm are moving forward. You're looking for a score of 2+ to be considered normal.

- ✔ **White blood cells:** Too many white blood cells can indicate an infection in your groin. A passing grade is no more than 0 to 5 per power field.

- ✔ **Hyperviscosity:** Your semen sample should liquify within 30 minutes after ejaculation. If it takes longer, it reduces the chances for sperm to swim before being expelled from the vagina.

- ✔ **pH:** Like an AA battery, your semen needs to be alkaline in order to avoid making the vagina too acidic and, ultimately, killing the sperm.

In addition to the above, a semen analysis evaluates the following:

- ✔ **Head quality:** The head of the sperm contains all of the genetic material, so if the head is misshapen, it won't be capable of fertilising an egg.

- ✔ **Midsection malaise:** Believe it or not, this part of your sperm contains fructose, which gives your sperm energy to swim. Low levels of fructose can account for slow swimmers.

- ✔ **Tail troubles:** Much like a fish, a good tail is required for the sperm to swim forward. If too many of your sperm have no tail, multiple tails or tails that are coiled or kinked, they won't reach their destination.

A low sperm count may have you feeling, well, downright low. Feeling embarrassed is completely natural but also completely unnecessary. Infertility has no correlation to a man's masculinity, nor does it have anything to do with the size of his penis. Having a low sperm count is no different to having asthma – it's a medical condition that requires treatment.

Identifying and treating the causes

Because sperm counts are created months before the sperm are used, you'll need to have a follow-up semen analysis to see if the issue is corrected by lifestyle changes. Although you won't be in a rush to do it all again anytime soon, whether your results are good or bad, schedule a follow-up analysis four to six weeks after the first one to get a better, more complete picture.

The most common cause of a low sperm count is a *varicocele*, an abnormality in the vein in your scrotum that drains the testicles. Varicoceles can cause decreased fertility in the following ways:

- ✔ Increasing temperature in the testes.

- ✔ Decreasing blood flow around the testicles.

- ✔ Slowing sperm production and motility.

Varicoceles are treatable in the following ways:

- ✔ **Surgery:** A simple outpatient procedure during which an incision is made just above the groin and the swollen vein is 'tied off'. Recovery takes seven to ten days and requires minimal activity and no heavy lifting. Risks are minimal but include infection, nerve injury and the collection of fluid around the testicles.

- ✔ **Radiographic embolisation:** This requires the insertion of a catheter through the femoral vein in the groin. Dye is injected to show where the problem is located and, when isolated, the vein is blocked so blood flow to that vein stops.

Other, less common, male fertility issues include the following:

- ✔ **Hormone imbalances:** Medications to adjust hormone levels may improve sperm quantity.

- ✔ **Chromosomal abnormalities:** One such problem is sperm that lack part of the Y chromosome, the male chromosome. *In vitro fertilisation* (IVF) and *intracycloplasmic sperm injection* (ICSI), where the best-looking sperm are injected directly into your partner's egg in the lab, can help overcome abnormal sperm issues. (See the following section for more info.)

- ✔ **History of cancer:** Having treatment for cancer, including lymphoma and testicular cancer, can kill or damage sperm. Many men freeze sperm before undergoing cancer treatment for this reason.

- ✔ **Various diseases:** Diabetes, sickle cell disease, and kidney and liver diseases can cause problems. Treatment depends on your individual issues.

Even if your ejaculate has no sperm at all, a procedure called a *sperm aspiration* in conjunction with an IVF cycle may be able to remove sperm directly from the testicles.

Deciding how far to go to get pregnant

Deciding what steps you're willing to take in order to get pregnant will be easier after you have a better understanding of the infertility issues you and your partner are facing. The most common procedures to aid in pregnancy are the following:

- ✔ **Intrauterine insemination (IUI):** A lab technician takes your sperm sample, pulls out the best of the best and adds it to a saline solution, which then is inserted past your partner's cervix. This gives the sperm a far shorter distance to travel and a greater chance of success.

- ✔ **In vitro fertilisation (IVF):** Sperm meets egg in a lab, and then the fertilised embryo is placed into the womb. Fertilisation can take place by either placing a concentrated semen sample in a dish with the egg or via intraycloplasmic sperm injection (*ICSI*). In ICSI, a single sperm is injected directly into a mature egg. Even with ICSI, fertilisation may not occur, because the egg or sperm may be chromosomally abnormal, which in some cases isn't evident just by looking at it.

Try not to make too many long-term decisions about how far you're willing to go, because undergoing fertility treatments is like riding a roller coaster, and once you're on, it becomes harder to get off. Especially when it feels like your baby could be just around the next corner. Make decisions month-to-month and procedure-to-procedure to avoid stress and allow for an open, ever-changing dialogue with your partner.

Sharing Your Decision to Have a Baby

Deciding to try to have a baby is a very big, very exciting step for most couples, and increasingly it is something many people choose to share with a select group of friends and family members. News of an expanding family is usually met with joy, cheers and even a few inappropriate jokes about your sex life. But although sharing good news is fun, you also need to be prepared for people in the know to ask nosy questions and offer unwanted advice.

Considering the pros and cons of spilling the beans

Sharing the news means that you're turning your quest to have a baby into a mini-reality show that your loved ones are going to closely follow. Having a well of support during this time can be great, but having your mum and dad hinting for information every time you talk on the phone can also feel intrusive.

If getting pregnant takes longer than expected, you're also setting yourself up to have to deal with the inevitable questions about the delay. On the plus side, if you and your partner must deal with infertility, you'll need all the support you can muster.

Just make sure you're both ready to continue sharing information and dealing with questions from the people you tell. Once their curiosity is piqued and their excitement sparked, there's no turning back. (Especially for a first-time grandmother-to-be.)

Handling unsolicited advice about reproduction

You may think you've got a handle on lovemaking, but after you announce to the world that you're trying to have a baby, it may seem like all the people in your life suddenly become instant baby experts.

Now that reproduction is fodder for morning TV programmes and countless blogs and Internet sites, more people have more soundbites and nuggets of wisdom to offer you and your partner than ever before. If your mother tells your partner she shouldn't be eating that beefburger because she heard someone on the radio say so, or tells you that you really should be wearing boxers instead of briefs, you may find yourself at your wit's end before you even make it to the bedroom.

If your loved ones start interfering or offering advice that you don't want, thank them for their excitement and interest, but reassure them that you have the situation under control. Remind them that people have been having babies forever and let them know that being bombarded with all this information, be it from them, the TV or the newspaper, stresses out you and your partner, and that can decrease your chances of conception.

Not all unsolicited advice is about the act of having sex. Some people may think you're too young or too old to have kids. Your parents may chime in about how expensive kids are, implying that you're not financially ready to have a baby. Perhaps your stressed-out brother (and father of three) tells you to enjoy your freedom while you still can.

Whether somebody thinks you're too immature to be a father because you still play Xbox or that your partner's job is too demanding for her to be a mother, remember that the only voices that matter are yours and your partner's.

Part II
Great Expectations: Nine Months and Counting

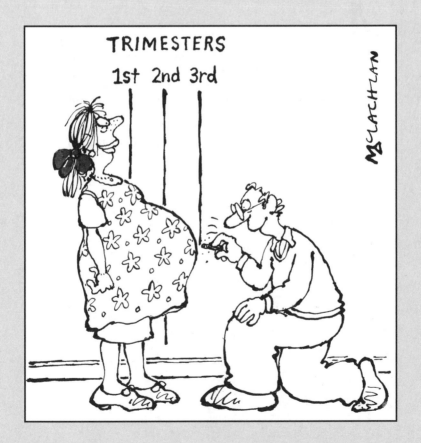

In this part...

*A*fter you've got past conception, a whole new field of emotions, experiences, and concerns pops up. From the sometimes uncomfortable moments of early and late pregnancy to the thrills of hearing the baby's heartbeat and seeing the first ultrasound pictures, pregnancy is a rollercoaster ride like no other. This part takes you from the positive pregnancy test to delivery options, covering every aspect of foetal and maternal growth as well as the all-consuming questions of what kind of stroller and car seat to buy.

Chapter 3

Surviving Sudden Doubts and Morning Sickness: The First Trimester

In This Chapter

▶ Getting the news that your partner is pregnant

▶ Attending important appointments

▶ Taking a look at foetal growth in early pregnancy

▶ Understanding the complications that can arise

▶ Taking on the role of a supportive partner

*F*ew new fathers-to-be actually pass out when they get the big news that there's a baby in their future, despite what you see on old television shows. That's not to say you may not feel a bit blown away by the news, though. Whether you've been trying for ten years or just met your partner last month, hearing that you're about to be a dad is life changing.

Early pregnancy is not without its physical, mental and emotional challenges, and although your partner bears the brunt of it, you can expect to experience a few symptoms, too. In this chapter we tell you what happens in the first few months and help you adjust to one of the biggest events in your life.

Baby on Board: It's Official!

Nothing is more momentous than hearing from your partner, 'It's positive! I'm pregnant!' If you've been trying to get pregnant for a while, these words are your cue to breathe a sigh of relief – your boys can swim! In fact, you may feel more relief than excitement at first. Trying to get pregnant can be quite stressful, as we discuss in Chapter 2, and the news that your worst fears can be put aside is reason for relief.

On the other hand, if this was a big 'oops' on your part – and many pregnancies are, even in this day and age – your first reaction may be more like, 'Oh . . . heck', or worse. Don't feel guilty if your first reaction is negative; most of the world's babies were an 'Oh, heck' at one time. In many cases, pregnancy takes time to get used to.

Reacting when your partner breaks the news

When your partner tells you the big news, try to mirror her reaction, at least outwardly. If her reaction is, 'Oh . . . heck', you can go along in that vein also, at least for a minute or two. Remember, though, that she's gauging your reaction to the news, and if you act like having a baby is a huge imposition in your life, she's going to be really upset, even if she just said the same things five minutes before.

So try to throw in a few encouraging statements about how you wanted kids eventually, having a baby will be fun in the winter when there's nothing else to do or whatever encouraging babble you can come up with at a stressful time.

Some women get very creative with their announcements, from filling the living room with balloons to baking a cake with a pair of booties inside. Just try to not choke on one, literally or figuratively. If she's gone all out to break the news, you can safely bet that she's really excited, so make sure she knows you feel the same way.

Even if you've been trying to conceive forever, an initial reaction of fear isn't uncommon. Remember that your partner may also be feeling some sudden doubts and fears, and allow her to express them. Under no circumstances is 'We spent £20,000 on fertility treatment and now you're not sure this is the right time?' the right response to her feelings of concern.

Making the announcement to friends and family

Deciding when to tell family and friends is tricky. On one hand, telling on the first day of the missed period makes the pregnancy seem about 15 months long, and telling early means you'll need to go through the grief of telling everyone if a miscarriage occurs, which happens in around 20 per cent of pregnancies.

On the other hand, you may have told people you're trying, and they may be obsessively counting the minutes until your partner can take a pregnancy test, too. If that's the case, saying, 'We don't know yet; we forgot to do the test' is going to make you look stupid and 'We've decided not to tell anyone' will probably get you thrown off the Christmas card list.

If you've already had to deal with a miscarriage, you may be understandably more reluctant to tell people in the first trimester. Nearly all miscarriages occur in the first 12 weeks of pregnancy, and most of those occur before 8 weeks, so waiting until you're pretty sure the pregnancy is going well may be prudent.

Whenever and whoever you decide to tell, realise that keeping news this big to yourself is hard. Even if you and your partner make a solemn pact not to tell a soul until after the first ultrasound, don't be shocked and disappointed to find out she's already told her best friend, sister and mother. In fact, she may have told them before she told *you*. Be understanding, and sheepishly admit you secretly told your parents, the guys at the gym and half your colleagues, too.

Overcoming your fears of being a father

You have a lot of time to get used to the idea of being a dad, so don't worry if you have a lot of fears at first. Even if you aren't sure you're ready to become a father, you'll be surprised at how quickly you come round to the idea. Besides, the baby will be here before you know it, ready or not.

When to tell work

For you, letting your work know that you're a father-to-be may not be such a big deal, because many workplaces still don't have any sort of paternity plan. If yours does, though, let your boss know after the first three months, when you're reasonably sure things will go well with the pregnancy.

If your partner is working and dealing with a lot of nausea or other pregnancy issues, the secret may be out earlier. The boss may not figure it out, but the rest of the workplace may.

It's important, however, to use this time to confront any fears about parenting that you may have. Spend time with the male role models from your past and present and use them as learning tools. Ask them what they did right, what they would change and what advice they have for you when raising your own child. It may feel like you're the first father ever, but you don't need to reinvent the wheel when it comes to parenting. If you admire someone else's skills, monitor and mimic their behaviours.

Working on overcoming your fatherhood fears is doubly important if the father in your life wasn't the best role model for the type of dad you want to be to your son or daughter. To attempt to come to terms with any wrongdoings your father may have committed, talk with a counsellor or therapist, or even a trusted friend, about your relationship with your father and try to identify the mistakes you don't want to repeat. Talking about your experience with your own father can also help heal some of the emotional wounds. Being a father is hard work, and you don't want to wait until after the baby arrives to start overcoming your fears or past traumas.

Attending the first of many antenatal visits

Many dads now attend antenatal visits, in stark contrast to the dark ages before 1970 when fathers never went near the obstetricians – or the labour room, either.

Everyone has a booking appointment around 10 weeks gestation. At this appointment you are counselled about screening investigations, including screening for Down's syndrome. The schedule of subsequent visits is not immovable but should occur every 4 weeks from the first visit to 28 weeks, then every fortnight from 28 to 36 weeks and then weekly until baby is born. At each visit, most or all of the following will occur:

- ✔ Blood pressure is checked.

- ✔ Weight is checked.

- ✔ A urine sample is tested.

- ✔ Blood tests (including a full blood count and those for blood group and antibodies, rubella antibodies, glucose, VDRL – for syphilis – and HIV antibodies, if you provide consent).

- ✔ Fundal height (the top of the uterus) is measured to see how well the baby is growing.

✔ The baby's heartbeat is monitored with an electronic Doppler device, which you and your partner can also listen to (this doesn't usually happen until 12 to 14 weeks).

Women who are *nulliparous* (who've never had a baby before) have appointments as outlined above. Women who are *parous* (who've had a baby before) are seen less often. In general, with a normal pregnancy nulliparous women are seen for ten appointments and parous women are seen for seven appointments

Going to the first ultrasound

An ultrasound scan is usually arranged following the first antenatal appointment. Some hospitals offer every pregnant woman two scans – one at about 12–14 weeks and another at 20 weeks, whereas other hospitals only offer one between 13 and 16 weeks. Ultrasounds are almost always done at the hospital and even though you won't see much, seeing that 'something' is in there is still a thrill! If you can get to this appointment, go.

Baby's Development during the First Trimester

When the embryo first implants in the uterus, about a week before a menstrual period is missed, it's too small to be seen without a microscope. Within a week, though, the first signs of pregnancy can be seen via vaginal ultrasound. While the embryo still isn't discernable, the gestational sac that surrounds him shows up as a small black dot. From this point on, foetal growth is an astounding miracle.

He may not look like much now, but . . .

In six weeks your baby embryo grows from a ball of cells to a recognisable creature, although the exact species is difficult to define. Following are the changes that occur in the first six weeks of pregnancy, which include the first four weeks, the time from the last menstrual period to the first missed period.

✔ **Week 2:** Egg and sperm meet, usually in the middle of the fallopian tube. The zygote formed by the union of egg and sperm drifts down to the uterus over several days.

✔ **Week 3:** Implantation occurs 7 to 12 days after fertilisation. There may be a small amount of *implantation bleeding* as the embryo burrows into the uterine lining.

✔ **Week 4:** The menstrual period is missed. A pregnancy test, which detects minute amounts of *human chorionic gonado-tropin*, or hCG, may be positive as early as week 4. On ultrasound, a small dark spot, the gestational sac, may be seen. The embryonic cells divide into two sections during this week, one that will become the embryo and one that will become the placenta.

✔ **Week 5:** The yolk sac, which nourishes the embryo before the placenta forms, may be visible next to the gestational sac on ultrasound. The embryo now consists of three layers that will develop into different areas of the body.

✔ **Week 6:** During this week, the embryo looks like a bent-over bean with a slight curve at the end. The heart is still a primitive tube, but a flickering heartbeat can be seen on ultrasound as blood begins to circulate. Arm and leg buds are sprouting, and the eyes, ears and mouth begin to form, although they're still a long way from a finished product at this point.

Amazing changes in weeks 7 to 12

Although few people would say, 'Yes, sir, that's my baby' by week 6, between weeks 7 and 12 the embryo really starts to look human (take a look at Figure 3-1).

✔ **Week 7:** In week 7, the baby is huge – around the size of a blueberry! At least he's something you could see with your own two eyes, and it's a 10,000-times increase over his original size. The brain and the internal organs are all growing, and the arms and legs have primitive hands and feet.

✔ **Week 8:** Fingers and toes start to form, and the nervous system is starting to branch out. Those new limbs are moving, although it will be weeks before your partner can feel movement, even if she swears she's feeling it already.

✔ **Week 9:** The baby's heartbeat may be audible using a Doppler, which amplifies sound. You'll never forget the first time you hear that rapid beat and realise there's a real human attached to it.

✔ **Week 10:** The kid doesn't even have knees yet, and he's already forming teeth in his gums! He does have elbows, though, and knees aren't far behind.

✔ **Week 11:** Your 2-inch (5-cm) bundle of joy is beginning to look like a real miniature person, one who has brand-new fingernails and an admittedly large head.

✔ **Week 12:** The internal organs are growing so much that they protrude into the umbilical cord (they'll start moving back into the abdominal cavity shortly), and the baby is making urine.

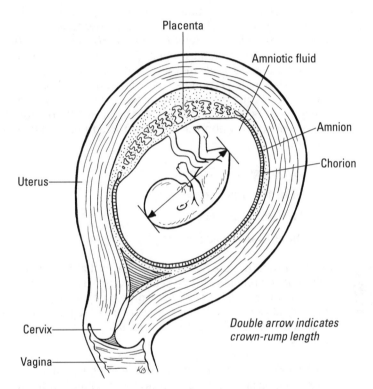

Figure 3-1: By the end of 12 weeks, the foetus actually looks like someone who just may be related to you.

Dealing with Possible Complications in the First Trimester

Although the majority of pregnancies really do go like clockwork, things can and do go wrong. In early pregnancy, the biggest threat is that of miscarriage. One in four women has a miscarriage at some point in her reproductive life. Another less common threat is an ectopic pregnancy. We discuss both miscarriages and ectopic pregnancies in this section and provide some tips for coping if you experience either of these complications.

Miscarrying in early pregnancy

Miscarriage is more common as women age, and though you may not consider your partner 'old' if she's older than 40, Mother Nature does, at least for childbearing purposes. In fact, doctors used to refer to pregnant women older than 35 as 'elderly'. The reason that miscarriage increases with age is that her eggs, which have been hanging around since before she was born, have aged, and you can't put face cream on eggs and have them look younger. The good eggs get used up first, so the ones left are more likely to be chromosomally abnormal. Miscarriage rates by age break down like this:

- ✔ **Under age 35:** 15 per cent
- ✔ **36 to 40:** 17 per cent
- ✔ **41 to 45:** 34 per cent
- ✔ **Older than 45:** 53 per cent

Keep in mind that these are averages and that a woman's actual risk depends on many other health factors. These numbers describe the potential risk *after* a pregnancy is diagnosed. Before the first missed period, many pregnancies are lost when they start to implant but then stop growing, usually because they're chromosomally abnormal.

The symptoms of miscarriage are bleeding that becomes heavier over time, passing clots and abdominal cramping. If your partner is newly pregnant, she may just have what seems like an unusually heavy period around the time of her period or shortly afterward. Pregnancies that end this early are often called *chemical pregnancies*.

Some women have spotty bleeding that isn't continuous, sometimes called a *threatened abortion*. (Abortion is the medical term for a miscarriage.) Some medical personnel still prescribe bed rest for women with spotting, although studies show it really doesn't change the risk of miscarriage.

The overwhelming number of miscarriages are caused by chromosomally abnormal embryos. You and your partner didn't cause the miscarriage, and you couldn't have prevented it. But although

miscarriage is a natural event, it's still an emotional loss (to vary-
ing degrees for different people) and talking about how you feel
is an important part of coping. Allow yourself and your partner to
mourn the loss of the baby, no matter how early in the pregnancy
it occurs.

Having one or two miscarriages doesn't increase the risk of it happening again, but women experiencing three or more miscarriages
should see a fertility specialist to determine the cause, if possible.
Following are some of the possible causes of recurrent miscarriage
(three or more losses):

- **Uterine abnormalities:** Fibroids, polyps, scar tissue or congenital uterine malformations can prevent the pregnancy from
  implanting properly in 15 to 20 per cent of recurrent miscarriage cases. Surgical correction of the abnormality may help.

- **Incompetent cervix:** An incompetent cervix dilates prematurely because it's been weakened by trauma or congenital
  deformities. Miscarriage usually occurs after 12 weeks.
  Incompetent cervices cause around 5 per cent of recurrent
  miscarriages and can be treated by placing a stitch in the
  cervix to hold it closed.

- **Chromosomal abnormalities:** You or your partner may carry
  genes that are causing recurrent miscarriage. Genetic testing
  can help determine the cause.

- **Immune system problems:** Women who have auto-immune
  disease can have recurrent miscarriages. Treatment with
  medication may reduce the risk of pregnancy loss.

- **Low progesterone levels:** Sometimes progesterone levels are
  too low to sustain a pregnancy, and supplementation helps.

After a miscarriage, many women pass all the tissue and need no
further medical care. Others need tissue surgically removed so
it doesn't cause infection or continued bleeding. This procedure,
called a *dilatation and curettage*, or D&C for short, is done as an
outpatient procedure.

If your partner passes tissue, save it and take it to your doctor
so he can see that everything's been passed and possibly test to
figure out what happened. When cramping intensifies, keep a clean
container with a lid in the bathroom so you can collect any tissue
as it passes. Take the tissue to your doctor as soon as possible;
keep the container in the refrigerator or follow your doctor's or
midwife's instructions on where to take it if a miscarriage occurs
over the weekend.

The miscarriage may be diagnosed afterwards as a *blighted ovum*, a pregnancy where the embryo stops developing and only the placenta grows. Blighted ovum is the most common type of chromosomally abnormal pregnancy. It can't be predicted or prevented; a certain percentage of embryos are chromosomally abnormal, and one blighted ovum doesn't mean the problem will recur in the next pregnancy.

Understanding ectopic pregnancy

Sometimes a pregnancy implants in the fallopian tube or, rarely, in another location, such as the ovary, abdominal cavity or cervix. A pregnancy that implants outside the uterus is called an *ectopic pregnancy*. Ectopic pregnancies are more common in women who have damaged fallopian tubes and occur in 1 in 100 pregnancies.

An ectopic pregnancy usually seems to be developing normally up until around seven weeks. An early pregnancy test is positive, but if an ultrasound is done, nothing shows up in the uterus. If the embryo is in the fallopian tube, the tube may appear distended.

If an ectopic is diagnosed early enough, medication to stop the pregnancy from growing can be given, which saves the tube or other implantation sites from being removed. The products of conception are absorbed naturally and don't need to be surgically removed if the drugs are given early enough and are effective.

Rarely, abdominal pregnancies have continued to the point where the baby reaches viability and can survive after delivery, but such cases are very rare.

When the ectopic pregnancy gets too far along, bleeding starts and the tube is in danger of rupture. At this point, removal of the fallopian tube is the only way to prevent serious blood loss that may threaten the mother's life. An ectopic pregnancy cannot be removed and replanted elsewhere, so the embryo will be lost.

Signs of ectopic pregnancy in danger of rupture include slight bleeding, abdominal pain on one side, lightheadedness, shoulder pain or passing out. Ectopic pregnancy is a life-threatening emergency. Get to the hospital immediately!

Coping with pregnancy loss

Losing any pregnancy can be devastating. Many people you tell won't make coping with the loss any easier either, with comments suggesting it was 'for the best' or that 'you'll have another one soon'. Many people don't really see early pregnancy loss as some-thing to grieve over and may not understand why it's hitting you or your partner so hard.

In fact, one of you may not understand why the other is taking it so hard, either. Whether you're on the same page or not, be respect-ful of each other's feelings and give yourselves time to grieve. Attending christenings, family gatherings with lots of kids running around or children's birthday parties can be very painful during this time.

Don't try to handle what you're really not up for. If your partner doesn't want to visit your sister's new baby right now, help shield her from this situation. Hopefully your sister will understand that this is a temporary event, not a permanent rejection of her and your new niece or nephew.

Common First Trimester Discomforts – Yours and Hers

Early pregnancy can be uncomfortable – for both of you. Though your partner bears the brunt of it, the first three months of preg-nancy may bring some unwelcome changes into your life as well. Hang in there, though – it'll all be worth it in the end!

Helping your partner cope with the symptoms of early pregnancy

Early pregnancy brings extreme fatigue and the overwhelming desire to take a nap, food cravings, food aversions, nausea, vom-iting and a constant need to urinate. Not to mention hormonal changes that cause pendulum-like mood swings, from crying to euphoria almost before you can ask what's wrong.

Knowing the symptoms ahead of time helps you keep your cool when all around you seems to be falling to pieces. Following are more things you can do to help your partner through these first topsy-turvy months of pregnancy:

✔ **Let her rest.** Although sitting at home all weekend watching her take two naps a day may not seem like a whole lot of fun, use this time to get projects done around the house or catch up on your parenthood reading.

- ✓ **Help her.** Shoulder some of her chores for now, especially the ones that make her nauseous, such as cooking, putting out the rubbish, dishing up the dog food and cleaning the toilet. Remember that handling cat litter is strictly off-limits for pregnant women (see Chapter 5), so that's your job, too.

- ✓ **Accept her limitations.** Maybe you went out to eat several times a week and now the sight of restaurants makes her sick. Hang in there. By the middle trimester she'll be eating everything in sight, and your favourite restaurant will still be there.

- ✓ **Don't take emotional outbursts seriously.** Not letting her outbursts get to you is hard when they're pointed at you and all your shortcomings, but listen to what she says, accept what may actually be true and disregard the rest. Don't forget to fix any shortcomings you can, though.

- ✓ **Satisfy her cravings.** Not that many pregnant women really want pickles and ice cream, but if your partner does, get some for her. Try not to gag as you watch her eat them; you may have to leave the room yourself.

- ✓ **Plan pit stops.** If you're the type of driver who doesn't stop the car unless the road abruptly ends before you reach your destination, realise that pregnant women really do have to pee every five minutes; she's not making up an excuse to go in to the petrol station for a bar of chocolate. Also, because blood volume increases during pregnancy, blood clots can develop if she doesn't move her legs regularly. Let her get out of the car every few hours!

Getting used to strange new maternal habits

At times, you may look at your partner and wonder who this woman actually is. The sweet-tempered woman you once knew may have been replaced by someone whose head appears to be rotating at times, and the woman who used to party all night long barely makes it into the living room to collapse on the couch after work. You knew having a baby was going to change your life, but you probably didn't expect things to change this much so early in the game.

Take heart: these are temporary changes. After her body adjusts to the new hormone levels, many of the symptoms will decrease, and your original partner will start to emerge again.

In the meantime, some of her new habits may be impacting on you in a big way, and you may need to find ways to cope with them. The following sections help you deal with a few of your least favourite early pregnancy things.

Vomiting

Although she's the one vomiting, sometimes you may not be far behind. Many people have a hard time dealing with vomit, whether it's their own or someone else's. If you have a sensitive stomach, hearing her heave may inspire the same reflex in you. Staying supportive while holding on to your own lunch can be difficult. You may want to try the following tips if the sight, sounds and smell of vomiting are getting to you:

- ✔ **Dab something under your nose that smells good to you.** Doing so really helps. Peppermint oil can get you through some tough moments. Nose plugs may also work, if your partner doesn't take offence at them. She probably doesn't want you to start vomiting too, so she may be okay with this new look.

- ✔ **Stay cool.** People are less likely to vomit when cool air is blowing on them, so turn the fan all the way up and also get a small fan that can blow right on you. This may help keep your partner from vomiting, too.

- ✔ **Avoid trigger foods.** If certain things really get to her, make sure they don't enter your house, no matter how much you crave them.

Gaining weight

While weight gain isn't such a problem during the vomiting weeks, when the nausea ends, your partner may start eating like food is going to be taken off the market next week. This can be bad for her waistline, certainly, but it can also be not so good for yours, since you may find yourself overeating just to keep up with her and matching her weight gain pound for pound. The woman who never let a chocolate-covered cake in the house may now be eating them by the shed-load.

For both of your sakes, try to put a stop to the madness. You don't have to remind her how hard this weight is going to be to lose later; just talk about your own weight gain and how you're afraid you won't be able to play frisbee on the beach with the kid if you keep eating like this. Don't turn into the food police; no one responds well to being told what they should and shouldn't eat.

Even if your pleas for healthier food choices don't get her out of the junk food aisle and back into the vegetable section, force yourself to cut back on the unhealthy foods. She's eating for two, but you aren't, although you may look like you are about halfway through the pregnancy. And, all kidding aside, that extra weight will interfere with your ball-playing and piggy-back-ride abilities down the road.

Coping with your cravings

If an active sex life was part of your semi-weekly (or more) agenda, you may be in for a rough few weeks. Sex may be the last thing on her mind in the first trimester. And some types of sex may trigger her gag reflex, which is the last thing you want to associate with a previously enjoyable activity! While turning into a monk may not be on your list of fun things, you can cope with the words 'Not tonight, darling' by

- ✔ **Experimenting with touching.** Depending on how open your partner is to experimentation, you can do a lot to pleasure each other that doesn't involve intercourse. In fact, this may be a great time to start understanding your partner sexually more than ever before. Find out what she's up for by taking it slow, working together to find comfortable positions and techniques, and by being supportive if at any moment she needs to stop.

- ✔ **Practising self-release.** Masturbation isn't something most adults like to talk about, but if you have a voracious sexual appetite and both you and your partner are okay with the idea, there's no shame in taking the matter into your own hands, so to speak.

- ✔ **Watching her patterns.** If morning sex used to be your thing but her new thing is promptly vomiting every time she wakes up, shake things up. Try to engage in sexual activity at times of the day when she's generally not tired, nauseous or weepy.

- ✔ **Being flexible – this too shall pass.** Some women are ready for sex sooner than others and, for some, when the sex drive returns, it's strong. It may come and go throughout the day. Be ready to perform when your partner is ready, because the window of opportunity can be slammed shut before you've even had a chance to look outside.

A desire to have sex is normal, and becoming frustrated during the time she isn't up for it doesn't make you a pig. Don't push the issue or make your partner feel bad about the lack of sex, but do let her know that you miss being with her and look forward to when she's up for having sex again. In the meantime, work off that extra steam with a nice run or a game of tennis.

Taking on your emerging support role

Don't think of yourself either as your partner's personal assistant or as the pregnancy police. She may become a diva in her pregnancy, but it's not your responsibility to do it all. And try to avoid becoming overprotective of your partner's physical capabilities, especially early in the pregnancy. If everything goes well with the pregnancy, she won't have many restrictions on her activities. But that doesn't mean she's going to be up for taking care of everything she's always managed.

For the first several months – and for the last few – your partner may be too tired/nauseous/hot/and so on to make dinner, walk the dog or perform many of the household chores you used to split. Pick up the slack until she feels good enough to contribute again. When she's back in the swing of things, she can move around and help again. Physical activity is beneficial for both mum and baby.

One of your main roles is ensuring that she eats healthily and exercises if and when possible, but the way to do this is by example, not with a whip and chain in hand and bathroom scales placed in front of the fridge. Ask her to take walks with you and help by preparing meals that will settle her stomach and feed baby's growing systems.

Pregnancy does not turn your partner into a child, even though she's carrying one around with her. She still gets to make her own choices about what she eats, and when or if she exercises, and you may have to bite your lip if she starts exceeding the weight limit for your delicate Queen Anne chairs.

In addition to supporting your partner physically, you need to support her emotionally. She'll probably be weepier and more sensitive than normal. If you're not the kind of guy who likes to talk about feelings, we suggest you become that guy for a month or so.

As hormones surge and wane, roll with the punches. Let the little things go without a struggle, because your partner won't always be able to control her reactions the way she used to. Let her dictate what's for dinner, and if her stomach turns when you present her with the exact meal she asked for, don't take it personally.

Being a rubber wall isn't easy, but the more you can let things bounce off you, the easier this time is for everyone. Supporting your partner throughout pregnancy is a constant game of choosing your battles and helping her make healthy decisions for her and the baby. Don't tell her what she should do – lead by example. Doing so is good practice for when you have a child in the house.

Chapter 4

Growing Into the Second Trimester

*W*elcome to the best three months of pregnancy, for both you and your partner. The second trimester is universally regarded as the 'golden era' of pregnancy – she's big enough to look pregnant and not just pudgy, morning sickness is left in the dust, and the aches and pains of late pregnancy are still in the distant future. Enjoy these three months, because the next three will bring much more upheaval into your partner's life – and consequently into yours!

In this chapter we walk you through the garden of the second trimester, with your first exciting look at your baby, finding out the sex (if you want to) and a few emotional upheavals.

Tracking Baby's Development during the Second Trimester

By the end of the first trimester, your baby's vital parts are all in place and beginning to perform the functions they'll carry out for the next 80 or so years. By the end of the second trimester, the baby's lungs, one of the slowest organs to mature, are almost capable of supporting life with assistance if she's born very prematurely (23 to 24 weeks is considered the earliest that a foetus can survive if born early). But the lungs aren't the only area experiencing change; every body system is becoming more refined with each passing day.

Growing and changing in months four and five

Even though the basic structures are in place, they undergo further refinement in months four and five:

- ✔ **Week 14:** The baby's eyes close for several months while they develop on the inside.

- ✔ **Week 15:** Some women may start to feel flutters when the baby moves; many women, especially those in their first pregnancy, don't feel movement for several more weeks.

- ✔ **Week 16:** Hair (including eyebrows) begins to grow.

- ✔ **Weeks 17–18:** Air sacs start to form in the lungs, but the lungs won't be able to support life for another six weeks or so.

- ✔ **Week 19:** The permanent teeth form in the gums. The baby can swallow.

- ✔ **Week 20:** By this week, the midpoint of pregnancy, the foetus is around 6.5inches (16.5cm) long and weighs around 10ounces (284g).

- ✔ **Weeks 21–22:** The foetus now has a functioning tongue! A baby girl's ovaries contain all the eggs she'll ever have in life, around 6 million.

- ✔ **Week 23:** The baby can now hear but, more importantly, if born now, she has around a 15 per cent chance of survival.

Figure 4-1 gives you an idea of what these changes look like.

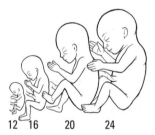

12 16   20   24

Figure 4-1: Months four and five of pregnancy.

Refining touches in the sixth month

The sixth month continues the refining process; all the major components are in place, and all the baby has to do is grow and mature.

- **Week 24:** Your baby has around a 50 per cent chance of survival if born at this point. She now weighs around 1.3 pounds (0.6 kg).

- **Weeks 25–26:** The spinal cord and lungs are forming more completely, and the eyes reopen at last!

- **Week 27:** At the end of the second trimester, your baby approaches 2 pounds (1kg) and 14.4inches (36.5cm). The lungs, spine and eyes continue their refinement process. Every week increases the odds of survival if born early.

Check out Figure 4-2 to see how much baby has developed by the end of the sixth month.

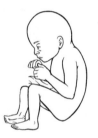

Figure 4-2: By the end of month six of pregnancy, the foetus is likely to survive if born early.

Checking Out Mum's Development in the Second Trimester

The middle trimester of pregnancy may be the best time of your partner's life: she feels good, looks 'cutely' pregnant and usually enjoys these three months, which means that you get to enjoy them, too! It's also the time when her sex drive may return and the urge to begin getting the home ready for baby kicks in.

During this time, make the most of your waning days as a twosome. Later in the pregnancy, your partner may not be up for doing as much, and after baby arrives all bets are off. So get out now! Go on dates, take a holiday or just indulge in all the things that you and your partner enjoy doing together.

Now is also the time when your partner's body goes through a lot of changes, which means that your support is more important than ever. Giving up her body for a baby isn't easy, and the more you help her deal with the ups and downs of pregnancy, the easier it will be for everyone.

Gaining weight healthily

One of the most overwhelming concerns for many pregnant women is weight gain. They're afraid they're gaining too much, aren't sure how much they should gain each month and are desperately afraid that extra weight will be with them for a lifetime.

It's not unusual for dads-to-be to begin packing on the pounds, too. Perhaps you also indulged in your partner's first-trimester cravings. Maybe she wasn't feeling up for those long walks you used to take after dinner, so you skipped them as well. If you're gaining weight right along with her, you may have some concerns in this area, too! The following information may help you help her (and yourself) deal with weight gain issues:

- ✔ After the first trimester, a weight gain of around 1 pound (0.5kg) a week is considered normal.

- ✔ Total weight gain, on average, should be between 25 to 35 pounds (11.5 to 16kg), with underweight women gaining a little more (28 to 40 pounds/13 to 18kg) and overweight women less (15 to 25 pounds/7 to 11.5kg).

- ✔ Pregnant women need only an extra 100 to 300 calories a day.

- ✔ The baby contributes around 8 pounds (3.5kg) to the total weight; amniotic fluid, placenta, breast tissue and an increase in uterine muscle each add another 2 to 3 pounds (1 to 1.3kg). The rest is stored fat and increased blood, each adding around 4 pounds (1.8kg).

Keeping the emphasis on eating well during pregnancy helps you and your partner ensure that baby grows well – and that your partner won't end up with an extra 40 pounds (18kg) after the pregnancy. Focus on eating plenty of fresh fruits, vegetables and healthy protein sources and limiting junk food, rather than focusing on the daily weigh-in numbers. Pregnancy is not the time to keep an obsessive weight chart; even if you fear that she'll never get back to her normal weight, rest assured that she most likely will.

Pregnancy is also not a time to lose weight or avoid gaining it, unless she's very overweight and is working with a medical practitioner. If she's really cutting down on food intake, she may need some help dealing with her fear of weight gain. Talk to her GP or midwife about how to handle the issue, because it's a pretty sure bet she'll take their advice over yours when talking about weight gain.

And remember, leading by example is always the best option. The healthier you both are during this time, the more likely you are to continue those healthy eating habits after baby comes. Don't wait to start living healthily until baby arrives, because it won't happen. Soon enough, it will be your responsibility to teach your child how to eat as well as you.

Looking pregnant at last!

One annoying aspect of early pregnancy for your partner is looking not quite pregnant enough and worrying that she looks pudgy instead of pregnant. Thankfully, by the end of the second trimester, most women definitely look pregnant, although if your partner is overweight, it may still be difficult to tell, something that may frustrate her no end.

The days of voluminous maternity wear are, for the most part, long gone, although most women will invest in a few pairs of maternity trousers with an elastic tummy and a few shirts either in a larger size than they normally wear or made of a stretchy fabric. Women who have to dress well for work will probably break down and buy actual maternity clothes so they don't look sloppy if their clothes are just overall too big for them or to avoid the skin-tight 'hey, I'm pregnant, look at my belly!' look that may be considered out of place in an office.

Many pregnant women (and pregnant celebrities, too) today do accentuate their bellies with tight T-shirts, hip-hugger trousers and bikinis. If you're extremely conservative, the 'let-it-all-hang-out' look may bother you.

WARNING! Approach your partner carefully with any suggestions as to how she should dress in pregnancy. Pregnancy hormones may be under control in this trimester, but they make an immediate reappearance under duress. There's really no nice way to say 'I hate the way you're dressed', so you may just need to keep your opinions to yourself.

Foods to avoid during pregnancy

In the second trimester, a pregnant woman's first-trimester distaste for food and often decreased appetite seem to vanish in the wind. Your partner may now seem to be eating anything and everything with gusto. Although a healthy appetite is good for her and the baby, pregnant women must avoid certain foods that can be harmful to the growing foetus or to their own health. Some of the listed no-nos aren't good for you, either, so you can stop eating them together.

Mercury can affect the foetal brain, nervous system and visual development. Most fish contain some mercury, but some have very high levels of mercury and should be completely avoided by pregnant women, including the following:

✔ Grouper

✔ Mackerel

✔ Marlin

✔ Orange roughy

✔ Shark

✔ Swordfish

The following fish also have high amounts of mercury, but fish from this group can be eaten up to three times a month:

✔ Halibut

✔ Lobster

✔ Tuna

Following are some other foods to avoid, or at least limit, during pregnancy:

✔ **Cold meats:** Cold meats may contain listeria, a bacteria that can cross the placenta and cause miscarriage.

✔ **Soft-serve ice cream/frozen yoghurt:** Listeria is also the concern here as the machines used to make the ice cream or yoghurt can be magnets for bacteria.

✔ **Imported soft cheeses:** Soft cheeses can also contain listeria if made from unpasteurised milk. Brie, Camembert, feta, Roquefort and Mexican-style soft cheeses should be avoided unless made from pasteurised milk.

✔ **Raw eggs:** Raw eggs can contain salmonella, a bacterial infection that can cause severe vomiting and diarrhoea.

✔ **Raw meat:** Raw meat can contain a number of harmful pathogens, including coloform bacteria, salmonella and toxoplasmosis, which can cause severe foetal complications.

✔ **Unwashed vegetables:** Unwashed vegetables can also transmit toxoplasmosis as well as salmonella.

You can try buying her a few articles of clothing that fit your image of what a well-dressed pregnant woman should wear. She may just wear them, if for no other reason than that she doesn't want to hurt your feelings!

Figure 4-3 shows the position of the uterus during the fourth, fifth and sixth months of pregnancy, as well as where you can expect it to go throughout the rest of the pregnancy. You can see why pregnancy gets really uncomfortable in the third trimester.

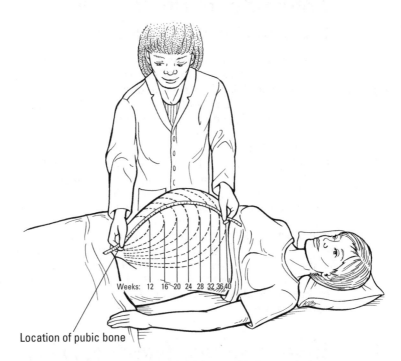

Weeks: 12 16 20 24 28 32 36 40

Location of pubic bone

Figure 4-3: Uterine height (the height of the womb) changes during pregnancy.

Testing in the Second Trimester

The second trimester is often the time for blood tests and ultrasounds that show the baby's development is on target and no major problems exist. Blood tests to assess the risk of genetic defects are usually done between weeks 11 to 13 or 15 to 20, depending on the tests being done, and screening ultrasounds, which look at the baby's major organs for anomalies and often can determine the baby's sex, are done around week 20.

Some babies are extremely reluctant to show their private parts on screen, so not all parents learn their baby's sex from an ultrasound. If you can't find out the sex of your child, don't stress about it. Buying gender-neutral clothing and nursery décor is easier than ever. Greens and yellows work for boys and girls, and you'll always have time to add touches of gendered colours after baby comes home.

Preparing for the risks of tests and ultrasounds

Having screening blood tests and an ultrasound done bring risks of a kind, as well as benefits. Neither procedure carries any significant physical risk to either mum or baby, but the procedures do carry a risk of finding out that something is wrong with the baby. This is knowledge some parents would rather not have.

Most parents prefer to know if the baby has problems so they can consider their options and prepare for potential difficulties, but others would not consider terminating the pregnancy under any conditions and prefer not to know. This is a personal issue that all parents have to consider for themselves.

If you're opting not to undergo testing, make sure that your partner's medical practitioners know about that decision. Be upfront about your preferences so that you don't feel pressured by anyone further down the pregnancy road. Most midwives will allow you to make special arrangements so long as they pose no risk to the baby or mother.

Understanding blood test results

Although some antenatal screening tests are for your partner's overall well-being and check for potentially harmful medical conditions, second-trimester triple- and quadruple-screen blood tests are aimed at determining the risk of genetic anomalies in the foetus.

Also used in conjunction with second-trimester ultrasound tests, quadruple screens help predict the risk that the foetus has Down's syndrome, trisomy 18 or neural tube defects such as spina bifida or anencephaly, where part of the brain is missing.

Quadruple screens test the blood for four things:

- ✔ **Alpha feto-protein, produced by the foetus:** High levels of AFP may indicate neural tube defects, abdominal wall defects or multiple pregnancy.

- ✔ **hCG, produced by the placenta:** hCG levels may be higher than normal in Down's syndrome pregnancies.

- ✔ **Oestriol, a form of oestrogen made by the placenta and liver of the foetus:** Oestriol levels are low in Down's syndrome pregnancies.

- ✔ **Inhibin A, produced by the placenta:** Inhibin A levels are elevated in cases of Down's syndrome.

Following up on the test results

Remember that first- and second-trimester blood tests are screening tests only. They do not diagnose congenital defects; they only indicate the odds that a congenital defect exists. The risk also varies with maternal age: the older your partner is, the more likely you are to have a child with a genetic defect, although the risk is still low.

If your partner's screening test comes back as abnormal, the most important thing to do is stay calm. An abnormal result only indicates a need for further testing. Try hard to keep both of you thinking positive until you have a clear answer on what, if anything, is wrong.

Although around 5 per cent of screening tests are reported as abnormal, only 4 to 5 per cent of foetuses with abnormal test results actually have Down's syndrome. This is a very small percentage, so remain optimistic; the odds are highly in your favour for a good outcome.

In the second trimester, *amniocentesis* may be done between weeks 15 and 20, when amniotic fluid is easily accessible. A thin needle is inserted into the fluid through the abdominal wall, and the foetal cells in the fluid are analysed. Amniocentesis comes with a slightly increased risk of miscarriage afterward, so most medical practitioners don't recommend doing an amniocentesis routinely.

Women older than age 35, who have a higher risk of having a child with chromosomal abnormalities, and those with a family history of genetic problems may consider having an amniocentesis, which can determine if chromosomal defects such as Down's syndrome, haemophilia, cystic fibrosis and other genetic disorders are present.

Scrutinising ultrasounds

As excited as you both are about the first antenatal ultrasound, the actual event can sometimes be a bit of a letdown. Reading ultrasounds is an art, and unless the ultrasonographer is really patient about pointing things out, you may be unsure of whether you're viewing the baby's head or its bottom.

Much depends on the direction the baby's facing. You may get a somewhat frightening straight-on face shot, which looks far more like a creature from *Dr Who* than any relative of yours, or you may get a front-on foot view that looks like nothing more than five round balls. You may be happy to know the baby has five toes on each foot, but that's usually not the main information parents-to-be want. The next section describes what the ultrasonographer is trained to look for.

Measuring growth

First and foremost, your medical practitioner wants to know that the baby is growing as she should. Some of the measurements taken to check for normal growth include

- The length of the longest leg bone, called the femur
- The head circumference
- The head diameter, called the biparietal diameter
- The abdominal circumference

Comparing these measurements to standards assures your practitioner, and you, that the foetus is growing as expected.

Checking for genetic markers

Genetic markers indicate an increased risk of congenital problems, but as with blood tests, genetic markers only indicate the risk potential; they don't diagnose the disease. Some ultrasound markers are known as 'soft' markers because they're often misinterpreted and not as diagnostic as other signs. Soft markers may also be transient and no longer seen in later ultrasounds. Following are genetic markers, including soft markers:

✔ **Thickness of the skin on the back of the neck:** Called nuchal translucency, thicker-than-normal neck skin indicates an increased risk of Down's syndrome.

✔ **Cardiac defects:** Around 50 per cent of Down's syndrome babies have cardiac defects, which may be visible via ultrasound.

✔ **Bowel abnormalities:** Around 12 per cent of Down's syndrome babies have gastrointestinal defects that may also be spotted on ultrasound.

✔ **Shortened arm and leg bones:** Children with congenital abnormalities often have arms and legs that are shorter than normal.

✔ **Missing nasal bone:** Failure to see the nasal bone or a shortened nasal bone on ultrasound may indicate Down's syndrome.

✔ **Polyhydramnios:** An increased amount of amniotic fluid may be associated with congenital defects.

✔ **Kidney abnormalities:** Dilated kidneys, missing or small kidneys and other anomalies may indicate genetic disorders.

Determining the sex by ultrasound . . . or not

While the ultrasonographer's priority is looking for information that shows the baby is growing properly, your consuming interest during the first antenatal ultrasound may be the baby's sex. In fact, the first scan is at ten weeks, which is too early to determine sex: the second scan is usually when you can tell. Ultrasonographers who do antenatal ultrasounds are well versed in not blurting out the sex of the baby and usually ask if you want to know. Most generically use *he* or *she* to avoid calling the baby *it* if you don't want to know, so don't assume anything by the choice of words if you've requested that you not be told. You can feel legitimately concerned if she starts using the term *they*, though! Ultrasounds are generally not done just to satisfy parental curiosity, but rather to catch any potential problems early on.

If you had your heart set on a girl and it's as plain as the nose on your face, even to your untrained eyes, that a little boy is on the way (or vice versa), remember that it's normal and okay to feel a twinge of disappointment. Try to keep it to yourself and concentrate on what you're probably seeing – a healthy, normally developing child.

If one of you really wants to know and the other doesn't, sort out a strategy before the appointment so that you're not arguing in front of the ultrasonographer. One method of keeping the news to just one person is to have the ultrasonographer write down the sex and put it in an envelope. That way, one of you can look and find out, and the other person doesn't have to.

This tactic also works if neither of you want to know at the moment, but you're concerned that your curiosity may get the better of you later. If you have the answer, you can look at it any time, but you don't have to.

Having Sex in the Second Trimester

For many women, the libido is back on the ascent during the second trimester, which will be a big relief for any guy who has patiently waited through nausea, exhaustion, discomfort and a lack of sexual energy for some long-awaited sex. In fact, some women become very sexual during this time because they're flush with hormones and feeling in touch with their bodies.

Maintaining a healthy sex life during pregnancy

Forget what you may have heard – sex during pregnancy is safe as long as your partner is having a normal pregnancy. Her desire to have sex may change by the day as the result of fluctuating hormones, tiredness or body aches. She also may struggle with being a sexual being as she transitions into the role of mother.

The most important thing to do is to keep talking about sex. As you get back into the swing of things, be open and honest about what you both need. Explore ways to satisfy each other's romantic and physical needs, even if your partner isn't up for sex.

Don't be surprised if your partner needs to take it slowly in the beginning. Stop at any signs of discomfort. As the baby bump continues to expand, you'll likely find yourselves exploring new positions that offer support for your partner's stomach. Many women are most comfortable on their sides or even up on their knees, and can use pillows for stomach support.

If your partner desires oral sex, it is absolutely safe. Just make sure not to blow air into the vagina because doing so can cause an embolism (a blood clot), which can be fatal for the baby and the mother-to-be.

Addressing common myths and concerns

We'll just get the myths out of the way right now: your penis is not long enough to hit or poke the baby during sex. The baby cannot see your penis when you're having sex, and she isn't afraid of your penis during sex. Your semen will not get all over the baby upon completion of sex.

Sex is perfectly healthy during pregnancy. Your baby is protected by an amniotic sac that's sealed tightly by a thick mucus plug, which keeps out foreign and unwanted intruders. In a few instances, however, sex during pregnancy isn't recommended. Talk with your partner's doctor or midwife prior to having sex if your partner has experienced any of the following:

- ✔ **Miscarriage:** If your partner has ever had a miscarriage, or a medical professional has said she is at risk for having one, check before sex.

- ✔ **Bleeding:** Sometimes vaginal bleeding ranging from normal to potentially life threatening can occur during the early months of pregnancy. Sex can cause the cervix to bleed, which can be alarming if you're already worried about bleeding.

- ✔ **Premature labour:** If your partner gave birth to a previous child prematurely, check with her medical practitioner to make sure having sex is safe.

- ✔ **Leaking amniotic fluid:** Any time amniotic fluid is leaking, the sterile barrier between the baby and the outside world is broken, and infection can enter into the uterus and infect the baby. No sex after her water breaks!

- ✔ **Placenta praevia:** With the placenta close to or overlying the cervix in placenta praevia, having sex can cause life-threatening bleeding.

- ✔ **Weakened cervix:** Sometimes called an *incomplete cervix*, this condition means the cervix dilates before full-term, which can lead to miscarriage. A stitch is often placed into the cervix to keep it closed. Sex can cause uterine contractions that disrupt the stitch.

- ✔ **Being pregnant with multiples:** Because multiples often deliver early, you need to avoid anything that can upset the delicate balance between no children and two – or more – children, sex included. Semen contains substances that may bring on labour if the tendency for premature delivery exists. Besides, your partner probably has enough going on in there already.

A female orgasm during low-risk pregnancy will not cause your partner to go into labour prematurely. Contractions of the uterus associated with sex are not the same as those experienced during labour (and your partner is *very* thankful for this!). However, orgasm achieved by any method can start contractions that can lead to premature labour in high-risk pregnancy, so put the vibrator away for the duration as well.

Some doctors recommend avoiding sex during the final weeks of pregnancy because of the prostaglandins in semen, which are hormones that can stimulate contractions. On the flipside, if your partner is overdue, your doctor may 'prescribe' sex as a means to jump-start the contractions.

Exploring Different Options for Childbirth Classes

You may want to attend childbirth classes as well as your partner's antenatal appointments. The good news is that lots of classes are available that are welcoming to both mother and father. And they aren't just about learning how to breathe! These classes are an opportunity to ask questions, build confidence and connect with other couples going through the same experiences.

Regardless of the type of class you sign up for, you'll be shown the basics in the following areas:

- ✔ Techniques for coping with labour and delivery pain.
- ✔ Your role in assisting your partner.
- ✔ What labour feels like/signs of labour.
- ✔ How to choose the birthing option that's right for you and your partner.

Selecting the class that's right for you has a lot to do with the kind of childbirth experience you and your partner want to have. Whatever class option you select, meet with the instructor prior to signing up to make sure he or she is the right teacher for your needs. Ask what's covered in the class, how many couples are in the class, where the class is held and for how many weeks the class runs. A fee is usually charged for attending these classes and booking them sooner rather than later is a good idea since they're in high demand. Provision of these courses varies from area to area, so finding out early in the pregnancy what's available and how soon you need to book is worthwhile.

Following are the most popular types of classes offered:

- ✔ **National Childbirth Trust (NCT) classes:** Run by highly trained teachers, these classes prepare you to make informed choices about what you would like for you and your baby (www.nct.org.uk).

- ✔ **HypnoBirthing:** Sometimes called the Mongan Method, this class teaches couples how to use relaxation and visualisation – self-hypnosis – to have a natural, intervention-free childbirth when possible (www.hypnobirthing.co.uk).

- ✔ **The Alexander Technique:** These classes focus on utilising techniques that reduce tension in the body and offer the mother-to-be freedom of movement during childbirth (www.alexandertechniquesociety.com).

Chapter 5

The Fun Stuff: Nesting, Preparing and Naming

*A*s the calendar inches closer to baby's arrival, usually around month five of the pregnancy, many soon-to-be parents get the urge to bring order to the home. What may start as getting the nursery ready often triggers an avalanche of do-it-yourself projects and more items added to the ever-growing 'essential kit' list.

And to make this whole baby thing even more real, this is the time to think about names. In this chapter we tell you how to get through the planning and preparing without any major blow-ups!

Preparing the Nursery and Home, or 'Nesting'

Put down the twigs and leaves – it's not that kind of nesting. This nesting is all about making the concept of baby a real thing in your everyday life.

Nesting can give you a sense of progress in the seemingly endless pregnancy and serves as the first of many acts of giving and loving that you will show your baby. It can also be a great motivator for finally getting the kitchen cabinets repainted and replacing that broken bathroom tile.

Making the house spick and span – and then some

For many pregnant women, the biological need to nest can be powerful. It can also veer into the seemingly irrational as your partner donates to charity or bins perfectly good sheets, rugs and towels because they may have unseen germs. Some women even get the urge to grab a toothbrush and some disinfectant and literally scrub the house from top to bottom. This behaviour is perfectly normal.

Try your best to be supportive without breaking the bank on unnecessary purchases. If your towels aren't in need of replacing, suggest having them professionally cleaned instead. Sometimes, however, the best thing to do when your pregnant partner is going through a bout of nesting-induced hysteria is to just let her do it. It's a natural process, and, as with all things, this too shall pass.

However, don't just sit back and watch. She may not ask, but she definitely wants you to help with the cleaning and organising. Even if you don't think everything she's doing is necessary, she may be unable to see why it's not as important to you as it is to her. Simply ask her how you can help or just join in with the express knowledge that this is a fleeting phase of late pregnancy.

This is also a time when your partner feels the need to launch a new set of rules regarding safety and cleanliness, such as no more shoes in the house or no more dogs allowed on the sofa. If your partner feels very strongly about something you disagree with, work together to find a compromise.

Some pregnant women are so bothered by the idea of pet hair, cat litter and the suspect grooming habits of animals that they may start talking about re-homing the family pet. As best as you can, try to delay any decision-making regarding your pet's future until after baby arrives. Hormones change following pregnancy, and the last thing you want is a crying partner feeling guilty about giving up Rover in the heat of the moment. Offer to take over the duties of pet maintenance for the remainder of the pregnancy and re-evaluate monthly.

Pregnant women have to be a little more cautious than normal while doing work around the house. Take note of the following household projects and their do's and don'ts:

> ✔ **Painting:** Pregnant women should avoid the urge to paint the nursery – or any wall, for that matter – because among other potentially harmful chemicals, latex paint may contain mercury, and old paint may contain lead; both of which can cause

birth defects. Sanding and breathing in particles are also a no-no. If your partner is going to be around while you coat the walls, make sure the room is well ventilated and that no food or beverages are consumed in the room where you're painting.

✔ **Cleaning:** Using eco-friendly cleaning products is always better, so start during pregnancy. Not only will your partner avoid exposure to harsh chemicals, but you'll already be pre-pared for the day when baby is crawling around and putting everything in his mouth.

✔ **Lifting:** It's a myth that lifting heavy objects lowers a baby's birth weight or causes birth defects. (Also, raising her hands over her head doesn't cause the baby to become tangled in the umbilical cord.) But a woman's centre of gravity changes as her stomach grows and her tendons and ligaments soften. Lifting objects heavier than 25 pounds (11kg) in the last few months of pregnancy can throw her off balance and result in a fall, so have her leave the heavy lifting to you.

✔ **Pet care:** Pregnant women should not clean a cat's litter tray because of the risk of toxoplasmosis, a parasite in cat faeces that can cause congenital defects in the baby. To further decrease the chance of toxoplasmosis, make sure you clean the litter tray frequently, keep your cats indoors and avoid adopting new cats during pregnancy.

Setting up the nursery

Fun *should* rule the day when it comes to setting up the nursery, but overanxious parents-to-be often try to tackle too much at once. Begin your nursery designing with a planning session. Draw a bird's-eye floor plan of the room and start filling in the space with all the things you need. Decide on the placement of all the furni-ture and, before you run out and start buying, measure the allotted spaces to make sure you don't end up with a cluttered area.

Clearing and painting the room

Unless you're starting with an empty space, the next step is to empty the room and find a home for all of your displaced things. This chore is the least fun, but don't put it off. Having an organ-ised room just for your baby will make you feel less anxious about bringing him home.

When the room is empty, painting is a cinch. Since pregnant women shouldn't paint, this is your job. If you don't have the time or desire to paint, find a friend, family member or local painter to do it for you.

After the room is painted, have the carpets and rugs professionally cleaned, or refinish the floors if they need it.

Buying and assembling the furniture

When the paint is dry and the floors are ready, it's all about shopping and assembly.

Plan some alone time for assembly if possible. Cots often come with instructions that seem to be written in Swahili, and they don't just pop together. They're solidly constructed, which is good for baby's safety but bad for your frustration threshold. Take your time and figure on spending a few hours on assembly. Lay out all of the parts and read through the instructions (yes, actually read through the instructions!).

Most of today's instructions offer picture-only guidance, which can be quite vague and frustrating. If you can't understand what you should do based on the manufacturer's illustrations, don't just do what you think should be done. Take the time to call. Not only is the safety of your child at stake, but your warranty, too!

Assemble the cot in the nursery because many cots are too wide to fit through doorways, and believe us – you'll be very frustrated if you have to take it apart and do it all over again!

Opinions differ on _bumpers_, the quilted bands that are strung around the bottom of the cot. The Canadian government discourages their use because of the chance of suffocation, and a 2007 study in the US _Journal of Pediatrics_ determined them to be unsafe. The NHS recommends that they should not be used because of the risk of babies overheating, or becoming entangled. Others believe that with the use of a cot positioner, which keeps baby sleeping on his back, bumpers cause little increased risk.

Whether or not using a bumper is worth the risk is up to you and your partner, but it is a risk. If you use bumpers, make sure you remove them if you notice your baby creeping toward the bumper in his sleep. Another option is to use mesh bumpers, which aren't padded but do offer a breathable barrier between baby and the cot's bars.

Some parents opt to use _co-sleepers_, which are small, three-sided cots that lie right beside your bed, keeping the baby very close at hand. This arrangement is ideal for late-night feeds but less ideal when considering the amount of personal space you have to sacrifice.

Arranging the nursery for two or more

Not all nurseries accommodate just one little baby. Whether welcoming multiples or adding a second child into a pre-existing nursery, creating a space that works for more than one takes a little extra effort.

Multiples

The only real challenge in accommodating multiples is making room for them to sleep. Changing tables, dressers and cupboards can easily be shared when you invest in cupboard organising systems to allow more items to be stored in less space.

For twins, some people opt to use a single cot with a cot divider that literally splits the bed down the middle. This arrangement is great for space-limited parents, and research shows that twins sleep better when placed near one another as they were in utero. However, cot dividers are only a short-term solution because as the babies grow, each needs more space.

If money and space allow, you have many options for twin cots that are smaller versions of full-sized units and are generally built side-by-side. And if you're having more than two, you may want to look into bunked cots, which offer an individual space for each baby. Most are not notably stylish, but if you're having more than two babies, stylish cots are probably the least of your worries.

Older child and newborn

If you're going to have an older child cede space to the newborn, the situation won't be all that different from having multiples. Most of your work concerns maximising storage space with cupboard organising systems, baskets and bins. However, investing in a co-sleeper (a three-sided cot that attaches to the side of your bed) or a travel cot can be a lifesaver when the older child and the baby aren't on the same sleep schedules. And if your older child is still a baby, the travel cot also provides a secure place for him when you're tending to the newborn.

Baby-proofing basics

You have some time before baby starts getting into things, but that doesn't mean that the nesting period isn't the perfect time to baby-proof. In fact, doing it early allows you plenty of time to adjust to the complicated life of cupboard locks, plug covers and doorknob locks.

To make sure your baby is safe, take the following precautions:

✔ Get down on the floor, look at the room from baby's level and clear all potential hazards.

✔ Install rubber stoppers at the top of doors to keep baby's fingers from being pinched.

✔ Remove rubber tips from doorstoppers at floor level because they're choking hazards.

✔ Instal baby gates in dangerous locations.

✔ Use plug covers on all plugs and sockets below waist level.

✔ Instal cupboard locks.

✔ Add a toilet-lid lock.

✔ Make sure all rugs and mats have slip-proof pads underneath.

✔ Add foam coverings to the edges and sides of sharp furniture.

✔ Apply doorknob covers to keep toddlers from being able to open doors.

✔ Find an out-of-reach location for pet supplies and the cat litter tray.

✔ Remove any toxic plants or chemicals that are within baby's reach.

✔ Put plastic covers on the bath taps to avoid head injury.

✔ Put your rubbish bins in an inaccessible place – to baby, not to you.

✔ Keep bags and purses off the floor.

Monitoring options

Baby monitors have come a long way in the past few years. Your options range from hi-def, flat-screen CCTV units to the classic walkie talkie-like models. If you live in a larger home, a CCTV monitor may make more sense to save you a lot of trips to the nursery to check on noises. Even in smaller homes, it can be useful to have a video screen to check if that little noise was a minor disturbance or something requiring your immediate attention.

Regardless of your choice, make sure that the unit you purchase can effectively communicate at the distance between the nursery and the other rooms of your home. Many monitors can now transmit up to 400 feet (120m).

When in doubt, move it or remove it. Get into the habit of looking for small items on the floor, closing doors, putting the toilet seat down and putting all potential choking hazards out of baby's reach. After years of not having to think about where you throw your keys, retraining your brain takes a while, so start now.

Understanding the Art of the Baby Kit-List

Buying stuff for baby isn't as easy as it sounds. Babies need a lot of gear, but they don't need everything, so you need to think through your particular wants, needs and style before you hit the shops or go browsing on the Internet.

Some parents-to-be first realise how unprepared to care for a baby they feel when forced to choose between different styles of bottles, nappies and baby monitors. Some couples enter panic mode and just start buying one of everything because they feel like their baby *might* need it.

The more online research you do about the differences between various products, the more competent and confident you will begin to feel about your parenting duties to come.

Doing your homework ahead of time to get exactly what you want

When you're thinking of buying the necessities for baby, everyone who has been a parent will tell you the things that you won't be able to live without. In truth, you *have* to have very few items in order to raise a baby, but a lot of modern inventions can make raising a baby easier.

First, consider your space. If your nursery is too small to hold an entire bedroom set and a rocking chair, you and your partner need to prioritise. The size of the room helps dictate the size and number of items you can add to it, as well as the style of cot, cupboard, changing table, curtains and every other accoutrement you can imagine. If you feel that a rocking chair is the one thing you must have, plan the rest of the room around that to make sure you have enough space.

A system for travel

Travel systems that offer a compatible buggy, infant car seat and car seat base in one package are a popular option for new parents. If you're on a tight budget, a travel system is an ideal solution to get everything you need for less than £200. However, many are quite bulky, and the included buggies generally aren't top-of-the-range quality.

Travel systems come in many styles, so start by picking the car seat of your choice. Make sure it has a five-point harness system and that it's the appropriate size for both your baby and your vehicle. Consider the size of the buggy too, and make sure it fits comfortably in your car boot. Make sure to collapse the buggy in the shop before you buy it to see how small (or big) it is when not in use.

 Get the essentials first and don't make your list too long, or you run the risk of not getting everything you need. Also, don't buy too many clothes because, although clothes are necessary, everyone will want to buy clothes for your baby!

 Spend time thinking about how you're going to use your pram or buggy. If you're a runner, do your homework about the best running buggies for you and try them at the shop. If you live in a city, make sure the buggy is durable enough to handle bumpy, uneven pavements, but not too big to make you the enemy of your fellow pedestrians. If you drive a lot, make sure the buggy folds up small enough to fit in your car and still leave room for shopping bags. And before you buy anything, check safety ratings and parent reviews online.

Finding out what you need – and what you think you won't need but can't live without!

When you've never before had to care for a baby, knowing what you need – and how many of each thing – is nearly impossible. Use the basic checklist in this section as your guide.

Note: We don't mention certain items, such as a highchair or play mats, because you don't need them right away. However, if you have room to store them, certainly pick the ones you want.

Remember, though, that when you meet your baby and get to know him, your idea of what he might like may change. The play gym you picked out before you met him may not really suit him.

Following are the items you absolutely must include on your list (in our opinion, at least).

Sleeping and changing essentials:

- ✔ Cradle/co-sleeper/cot
- ✔ Two to four fitted sheets
- ✔ Cot mattress
- ✔ Two to four swaddling blankets
- ✔ Nursery monitor
- ✔ Changing table or station
- ✔ Two to three changing-pad covers

Furniture:

- ✔ Nursery seating
- ✔ Baskets/bins for cupboard organisation

Clothing:

- ✔ Eight to ten babygros
- ✔ Eight to ten bodysuits (vests with poppers underneath)
- ✔ Six pairs of socks
- ✔ Three to six newborn hats
- ✔ Four to six warm, footed pyjamas or bodysuits
- ✔ Two to six bibs
- ✔ Eight muslin squares for burping and dribbles

Toiletries:

- ✔ Nappies (as many as you have room to store!)
- ✔ Wipes
- ✔ Nappy cream
- ✔ Baby powder

- ✔ Baby shampoo
- ✔ Baby lotion
- ✔ Hand sanitiser

Just in case:

- ✔ Digital thermometer
- ✔ Colic relief drops
- ✔ First-aid kit

On-the-go goodies:

- ✔ Infant car seat
- ✔ Buggy
- ✔ Backseat mirror
- ✔ Car window sun shades
- ✔ Nappy bag
- ✔ Portable baby-wipe container
- ✔ Travel-size hand sanitiser

Feeding:

- ✔ High-quality breast pump (if breastfeeding)
- ✔ Milk storage bags (if breastfeeding)
- ✔ Nursing pads (if breastfeeding)
- ✔ Lanolin and/or gel nursing pads
- ✔ Bottle steriliser
- ✔ Bottle brush
- ✔ Bottle drying rack
- ✔ One each of six different kinds of BPA-free bottles. (BPA is bisphenol-A, a chemical used in many plastics which may harm babies.)
- ✔ Four teats for each type of bottle

Not all babies take to every type of bottle; you may end up trying many different brands before you find the right one. Avoid buying too many of the same brand in case your baby refuses to use them.

Discovering three things you don't have to have but will adore

Yes, some things are luxuries, but they can become necessities if you use them every day and they save your sanity. These three items may well fit into your 'don't need it, gotta have it' category:

- ✔ **Ergonomic bouncy chair:** Not all bouncy chairs are created equal. Finding one that sits baby upright (great for wind relief) and allows him to grow with the chair will save you down the road – but not upfront. A bouncy chair is a perfect sanity-saver and a great place for naps and playtime for baby.

- ✔ **Hands-free baby carrier:** Whether in a sling, a front carrier or a pouch, carrying your baby in a hands-free carrier allows you to get work done around the house and move about more freely. Most babies love the body-to-body contact. Make sure to try them on first to make sure the carrier you're getting fits your body.

    Make sure you get a model that keeps the baby upright and able to breathe freely. When a baby slumps in a curled position, his airway can be compressed.

- ✔ **Yoga ball:** All babies get wind, and nothing helps get the wind out better than bouncing. Save your legs and back a lot of undue stress by sitting on a yoga ball and bouncing the burps right out of your baby. It's also a great alternative to a nursery chair for those with space limitations and a great late-term pregnancy chair for the woman who can't get comfortable.

Checking out five things you don't have to have and will never adore

Some things, luxurious or otherwise, are just downright unnecessary. Especially the items that don't actually make a new parent's life any easier. Here are five things you should consider omitting from your list:

- ✔ **Baby DVDs/CDs:** Before your child has the ability to ask for the latest album or DVD to be played ad nauseum, why on earth would you voluntarily spend your time engaging with this entertainment? Babies shouldn't be watching TV, and your child will be just as happy listening to music from your collection.

🖊 **Cot mobile:** It only takes one time of knocking into a cot mobile while putting your sleeping baby down to realise that it's more of a nuisance than it's worth. Instead, opt for a natural sounds teddy bear or other system that attaches to the side of the cot.

🖊 **Infant shoes:** If your child gestates for 18 months and comes out walking as nimbly as a newborn horse, you will need lots of fancy footwear. For the rest of you, forgo the shoes. Most babies are annoyed by socks, let alone shoes, and for the most part, babies under the age of six months will spend most of the time in babygros with attached feet.

🖊 **Car-charger bottle warmer:** If your baby is breastfed, the milk will most likely be frozen or straight from mum, and the warmer won't help. If your child is formula fed, you'll be making bottles as needed. Either way, how often will you need warm milk in the car? Most babies will be just as happy with room-temperature milk. Unless you plan on using it for your coffee, skip this one!

🖊 **Baby bath:** Why exactly does your baby need a smaller version of the same device you already have in your home? Many parents opt to bathe with newborns and most others use a clean sink in place of the tub. As baby grows, your existing bath will work just as well. Besides, it's not like you're going to give baby his bath-time privacy while you read the paper on the back patio.

Naming Your Baby

When people find out you're having a baby, the first thing they ask is, 'Is it a boy or a girl?' Question number two is inevitably, 'Have you chosen a name?'

Choosing a name for your baby is one of the most fun and most challenging decisions you'll ever make in your life. Soon-to-be parents spend hours upon hours combing through books and websites searching for the perfect name and making lists of their top choices. And with so many options, the list can easily become mind-numbingly long and a point of contention. Getting two people to agree on the same first and middle name for a baby can swiftly degenerate from a congenial conversation into something resembling a debate in Parliament.

The following section helps you and your partner choose the perfect name for your baby with as little stress as possible.

Narrowing down your long list

Just like a to-do list at work or that never-ending list of weekend projects you've been meaning to tackle for years, a long list of baby names will only distract and overwhelm you. Keeping the list at a reasonable length makes you more likely to engage in a meaningful conversation about the names that truly are in play.

 Remember that you're not really choosing between 30 names. Just because you really like all of them doesn't mean you don't like some more than others – you just may not realise it yet. Stop trying to choose between Jack, David, Ryan or Jude all at the same time. Instead, pit two names against each other at a time and choose one. This allows you to begin crossing some names off the list while continually pitting new names against the winner of the previous round.

At this point, you and your partner shouldn't take the opinions of others into consideration. The name is your choice, and unless you're ready to justify your choices, get frustrated with other people's input and stand up in the face of criticism, keep the contenders to yourselves until you've made a final choice.

Reconciling father/mother differences of opinion

In a perfect world, your favourite name is also your partner's top choice. The chances of that happening, however, are slim to none. When differences of opinion arise, don't get defensive. Be able to articulate why you like the name, and even do your research about the history of the name, the name's popularity and any family history regarding the name.

If your partner still doesn't like it, or you don't like a name she adores, allow each other absolute veto power. With so many names from which to choose, don't waste your time fighting a losing battle. And besides, do you really want your partner to cave in and name your child something she despises?

Discussing choices with friends and family

If you think talking about names between the two of you is hard, just wait until your loved ones start offering their ten pence worth. No matter what name you choose – be it classic, modern or something in-between – someone you know is going to tell you he doesn't like it. You'll probably hear it from multiple people, friends and strangers alike.

Don't feel the need to defend your choice. In fact, the more you defend it, the more likely the person is to continue to challenge you on your choice. Instead, focus on why you chose that name and don't be afraid to let other people know the matter is not up for debate. A playfully delivered, 'I guess it's a good thing this is my baby and not yours' can put them in their place without too many hurt feelings.

Even after the baby is born, the name will be under scrutiny. From your colleagues to cashiers at the supermarket, everyone will inquire about your baby's name, and you'll be confronted with a variety of reactions. Remember that people will have their own association with the name of your child, but at the end of the day, your only association with the perfect name you choose will be the perfect baby on whom you bestow that name.

Some people are reluctant to share baby names with others for fear that they may get 'stolen' by another friend or family member. If your partner has this concern and you do not, be very careful about sharing the name you choose. Though you may think keeping your chosen name secret is silly, she won't take it lightly.

Chapter 6

Expecting the Unexpected

● ●

In This Chapter

▶ Handling maternal medical issues

▶ Dealing with difficult ultrasound discoveries

▶ Knowing what to expect if baby comes early

▶ Managing multiple pregnancies

● ●

*Y*ou may assume that things will go off without a hitch during pregnancy and childbirth, but the fact is that many pregnancies experience some sort of complication. Complications may be related to your partner's health, the baby's well-being or to the pregnancy itself. Some complications are relatively minor, but others can pose a serious threat.

In this chapter we look at some of the things that can go wrong in pregnancy and guide you through to supporting your partner while dealing with your own fears.

Managing Pregnancy-Related Medical Issues

Problems that affect your partner's health sometimes develop with frightening speed. Other times problems develop insidiously and build to a crisis point. Neither is easy for a dad-to-be to deal with, especially when you have to keep your own fears under control so you can help your partner deal with hers. We take a look at some of the most common maternal pregnancy problems in the next sections.

Pregnancy-induced hypertension

Pregnancy-induced hypertension, often called PIH, is a newer term for elevated blood pressure in pregnant women. It is closely related to a long recognised disease, *pre-eclampsia*, also called *toxaemia*. PIH is elevated blood pressure that develops in 5 to 8 per cent of women after the 20th week of pregnancy. The signs of PIH are hypertension, retained fluid in the face and extremities, and protein in the urine.

Your partner is more likely to develop PIH if:

✔ This is her first pregnancy.

✔ She's older than 40.

✔ She had high blood pressure before she got pregnant.

PIH is dangerous because it reduces blood flow to the baby and also to the mum's major organs, including the liver, kidneys and brain. In severe cases of PIH, decreased blood flow to the baby can cause *intra-uterine growth retardation*, known as IUGR, which means low birth weight or stillbirth. Your partner may experience

✔ Severe headaches.

✔ Blurred vision.

✔ Light sensitivity.

✔ Abdominal pain.

✔ Decreased urine output.

New onset of any of these symptoms requires a call to your medical practitioner. Women with PIH often end up on modified or complete bed rest (see the 'Mandatory bed rest' section later in this chapter) or may at least have to stop working or work reduced hours. Resting on the left side increases blood flow through the placenta, and decreasing sodium intake can help lower blood pressure. Blood pressure medications may be prescribed if pressure rises too high. She'll probably need more frequent doctor visits and possibly more frequent ultrasounds to check on the baby's well-being.

Rarely, women with PIH need hospitalisation to control the symptoms and decrease the chance of eclampsia, which is severe PIH with seizures. Eclampsia can be life threatening for your partner and the baby and may require immediate delivery even if the baby

is premature. Part of your job is to watch for changes in your partner's mental state, such as confusion, irritability or disorientation,
because these changes may precede a seizure.

Gestational diabetes

Gestational diabetes, high blood sugar that develops during pregnancy and disappears after delivery, affects 2 to 5 per cent of pregnancies. Glucose testing for gestational diabetes is normally done
in the second trimester. Women who are diagnosed may be treated
with insulin injections to lower blood-sugar levels.

The problem with high blood sugar in pregnancy is that it
affects the baby, who will also develop high blood-sugar levels.
Gestational diabetes can affect the baby (and you) in several ways:

- ✔ The baby may grow larger than normal, which can make for
  a difficult delivery and increase the chance of a caesarean
  delivery.

- ✔ Babies whose mums have gestational diabetes are more likely
  to be born early and can have a severe and potentially dangerous drop in blood-sugar levels after the delivery.

- ✔ The baby may have to be monitored in the neonatal unit for a
  short time until her blood sugars stabilise, which is probably
  not the way you envisioned your time in the hospital.

If your partner is older than 35, is overweight or has a family history of diabetes, she's more likely to develop gestational diabetes.
Studies indicate that gestational diabetes is often a sign that she
may develop type 2 diabetes later in life.

The introductions of daily injections and monitoring can add a
whole layer of annoyance to pregnancy, for both you and your
partner. If she cooks, her cooking will probably become a whole
lot healthier, which you may or may not appreciate. If you're the
chef, you may be expected to devise a new repertoire of healthy
yet appealing meals. The bonus is that you both probably will be
healthier by the end of pregnancy if you follow her new diet.

Placenta praevia

Placenta praevia is a condition in which the placenta implants
too low on the uterine wall (see Figure 6-1). Usually the placenta,
which transports nutrients to the baby, implants near the top
of the uterus. If too low, all or part of the placenta can cover the
opening to the uterus, the cervix, and cause bleeding.

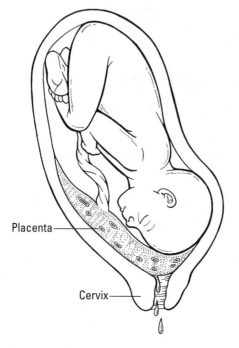

Placenta

Cervix

Figure 6-1: Placenta praevia.

 Bleeding from placenta praevia is painless, can happen without warning and can be severe enough to require immediate delivery. A known placenta praevia can necessitate bed rest and possibly a prolonged hospital stay to try to hold off delivery until the baby is less premature.

A marginal placenta praevia, one that's near but not covering the cervix, may allow for a vaginal delivery, but most of the time a caesarean will need to be done. And sex is out of the question, since anything that causes contractions or any cervical movement can start heavy bleeding. Your partner is more likely to have a praevia if

✔ She's had a previous caesarean delivery.

✔ She's older than 35.

✔ She smokes.

✔ She's of Asian descent.

✔ She's having more than one baby.

Setting up a bed rest station

Your bedroom may not contain all the elements needed to entertain a sometimes bored, often dejected woman who's just itching to get up and paint the nursery. But any space can be turned into a home inside your home, or inside the hospital, if necessary. Make sure her living space has all the following comforts:

✔ **A method of communication:** Unless your house is really small, yelling back and forth isn't the best method of communication. Walkie-talkies are great, and mobile phones work too.

✔ **A table to hold food and drink:** A drawer for snacks means she won't have to call for help every time she's hungry, and a coolbox filled with drinks by the bed also gives her a little independence. Some tables fit over the bed, but a table next to the bed works fine, too.

✔ **Entertainment:** A TV, books and magazines, cards, games, puzzles and a laptop computer all help pass the time.

✔ **Extra pillows:** Spending time in bed is really hard on your back, especially when you're pregnant! Invest in extra pillows to facilitate position changes. And take the Star Wars pillowcase off, too; give her something pretty and cheerful.

✔ **Space to work and something to do:** No, she can't load the dishwasher from the bed, but she'd probably love to fold baby clothes!

✔ **Pen and paper for shopping ideas and other thoughts:** She may see something on TV or think of something she'd like to try for dinner, so give her a way to write down ideas as they come to her.

✔ **Exercise ideas:** Even if she can't run around the bed, she needs to keep the blood flowing to prevent blood clots in the legs. Depending on what her doctor says is okay, encourage position changes, ankle circles and calf flexes several times a day. Discourage a cross-legged position, which decreases blood flow.

✔ **Venting room:** In this context, *venting* has nothing to do with fresh air and everything to do with letting her get frustrations off her chest. Constant negativity should be discouraged, but frustrated people need to express their aggravation, and better she vents to you than to her doctor – or her mother! So be available to her, not only to keep her company, but also to let her vent when she needs to.

Mandatory bed rest

If your partner has a risk of early delivery or other problems, your medical practitioner may put her on bed rest. Bed rest can mean anything from not going to work and taking it easy to not getting out of bed at all, even to go to the toilet, depending on the serious-ness of the medical condition.

Having your partner on bed rest is difficult for both of you. However, if bed rest is advised, take it seriously. Bed rest brings its own risks, mostly the risk of blood clots from inactivity, so doctors don't suggest it lightly.

And while bed rest may sound like fun, especially if you're running around trying to cook, clean, take the dog out, run errands and set up the nursery, trust us, she's not happy that she's unable to help put away the freshly washed clothes or hang the pictures on the wall.

Many women on prolonged bed rest get depressed, especially if they have to stay in the hospital rather than at home. Make sure to keep her in the loop of baby stuff; if it's okay with her doctor, get her friends to visit regularly. (See the nearby sidebar 'Setting up a bed rest station' for more ideas on helping her through the restric-tions of bed rest.)

Your partner's job is vital, though, and it's simple – stay put so the baby stays put for as long as possible. So make her feel like she's pulling her weight, because she is. In case you've never noticed until now, women often feel guilty even when they have no reason to. If your partner has to worry about how all the extra work is affecting you, she won't be resting peacefully, and staying calm and relaxed is essential on bed rest.

Handling Abnormal Ultrasounds

Many couples don't really relax about a pregnancy until they see the baby on ultrasound. But some couples don't come away from the ultrasound appointment with reassuring news. While ultrasounds aren't perfect and can miss some abnormalities, they recognise many problems.

In most pregnancies the ultrasound is done in the early part of the second trimester as by this time all the major structures of the baby are in place and can be evaluated. Ultrasounds may be done earlier if your partner is bleeding or if her doctor has any other concerns about the pregnancy. If anything suspicious is seen on ultrasound, then another ultrasound, done in the same way as a regular ultrasound but taking a more detailed look at the foetus, will be arranged.

Birth defects

Hearing that your baby has a problem is devastating. Even if a birth defect is minor, you or your partner may mourn the loss of the 'perfect child'. This reaction is normal, and neither of you should feel guilty. If a serious defect is found, you'll need to make decisions together about what to do.

Following are some of the most common birth defects in the UK:

- ✔ **Congenital heart defects:** 8 in every 1,000 live births.

- ✔ **Club foot:** 1 in every 1,000 births.

- ✔ **Down's syndrome:** 1 in 1,000 births; risk increases with age of mother.

- ✔ **Spina bifida (abnormal opening in the spine):** The most serious form of this, called a myelomeningocele, affects 1 in 1,000 births.

- ✔ **Anencephaly (lack of part of the brain):** around 1 in 8,000 births.

The most important thing to do when you get bad news is to find out exactly what you're dealing with. You may need to see a perinatologist, a doctor who specialises in complicated pregnancies, and possibly a genetic counsellor.

You and your partner may not be on the same page when it comes to making decisions about birth defects. One of you may be more optimistic about the situation and the other more pessimistic. Your feelings will be a jumble, and emotions will run high. Try to support your partner in whatever she's feeling, but don't discount your own feelings and grief, and don't feel like you can't let your feelings show. No one expects you to be emotionless at a time like this, and crying with your partner can be a bonding experience.

Expect to go through the five stages of grief: denial, anger, bargaining, depression and acceptance. Getting to acceptance can take a long time and a lot of anger. Give yourself the time you need.

Talking to someone outside the situation who listens and doesn't tell you what to do, like a friend, relative or religious advisor, can be a godsend. And most important of all, don't play the blame game. Congenital birth defects are rarely anyone's fault.

Foetal demise

Even more devastating than the discovery of birth defects on routine ultrasound is the discovery of a foetal demise. The term *foetal demise* is usually used to describe the death of the foetus in utero after 20 weeks. Many potential causes of foetal demise exist, and few if any can be anticipated or avoided.

Foetal demise may be discovered because the baby doesn't seem to be moving much, bleeding starts or amniotic fluid begins to leak, but it can also be found during a routine gynaecological check up. Foetal demise occurs in approximately 6 per 1,000 pregnancies overall.

Most foetuses are delivered vaginally after labour induction. Parents are encouraged to hold their baby and give her a name, but at no time will this be forced on you if you don't feel it's the right thing for you to do. Your partner will be given medication to dry up her milk supply and will be put in a room off the maternity floor in most hospitals. Most hospitals will let her go home as soon as she's physically stable.

In many cases parents are better able to get through a foetal demise if they know exactly why it occurred, but sometimes the reason isn't obvious. Not knowing why can be very difficult. Again, blame has no place in the aftermath of a foetal demise.

Preparing Yourself for Preterm Labour and Delivery

In England and Wales, 1 in 13 of all deliveries are preterm, which means they occur before 37 weeks. Of those

- ✔ 70 per cent are born between 34 and 36 weeks.
- ✔ 12 per cent are born between 32 and 34 weeks.
- ✔ 10 per cent are born between 28 and 31 weeks.
- ✔ 6 per cent are born before 28 weeks.

The chances of delivering a very small premature baby are low. Babies born between 28 weeks and term may require prolonged hospital stays, but most ultimately do well.

Recognising the risks of preterm delivery

Many preterm deliveries occur without any known cause, but in a good percentage of cases, doctors can pinpoint the reason. The following situations all increase the risk of preterm delivery:

- **Structural abnormalities:** An abnormally shaped uterus or an *incompetent cervix*, one that starts to dilate from the increased uterine weight, can cause labour.

- **Multiple birth:** A large percentage of twins, triplets and other multiples deliver before 37 weeks.

- **Infections:** Urinary tract infections can start uterine contractions if not promptly treated.

- **Hypertension:** High blood pressure can reduce blood flow through the placenta to the baby, causing poor growth that may necessitate early induced delivery.

- **DES exposure:** Diethylstilbestrol (DES) was a drug given to millions of women to prevent miscarriage between 1938 and 1971. Women whose mothers took the drug may have structural abnormalities that cause preterm delivery.

Handling feelings of guilt

Guilt is common after a preterm delivery, just as it is after any other setback in pregnancy. Again, don't get caught up in what you and your partner could have done to prevent it, or whose fault it is that you went for that long walk the day before the delivery. Even if one of you did something foolish, rehashing it now is pointless.

Put your energies into working with your partner to help your baby get healthy as quickly as possible. Visit often, and if support groups are available, get involved; studies show that parents involved in support groups experience less anxiety, anger and depression.

Navigating the NICU

The neonatal intensive care unit (NICU) is like nothing you've ever seen before. Although hospitals put more emphasis than they used to on keeping NICUs quiet and more like the womb, they are, by necessity, fairly noisy, with alarms going off, and the lights are on day and night so hospital personnel can see what they're doing.

At the centre of all this is your little baby. She may be hooked up to just a single monitor, or perhaps so laden down with medical equipment and IV lines that you can scarcely find the baby, as shown in Figure 6-2.

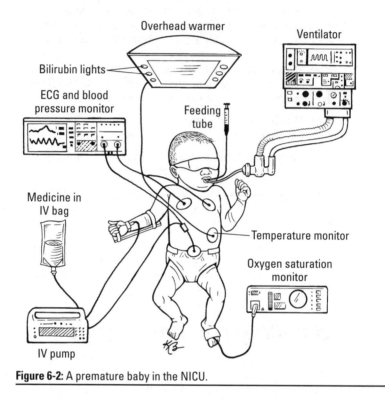

Figure labels: Overhead warmer, Ventilator, Bilirubin lights, ECG and blood pressure monitor, Feeding tube, Medicine in IV bag, Temperature monitor, Oxygen saturation monitor, IV pump

Figure 6-2: A premature baby in the NICU.

Focusing on your little part of this world is the best way to deal with the NICU. Get to know your baby's nurses, and stay in your own baby's area. Asking what's wrong with other babies is really bad etiquette, and the nurses won't (or shouldn't) tell you, anyway.

Many hospitals with large regional NICUs have facilities that allow parents to stay overnight for a small charge or for free.

If your partner is still in the hospital and can't see the baby right away, make sure you take lots of pictures, not just of the baby, but also of the neonatal unit and, if possible, of the people taking care of her. This way your partner can get a real sense of where the baby is and picture her in an actual place.

Expect the first time you hold your baby to be extremely awkward; she may be festooned in IV lines, and you'll probably be scared to death of her. Don't worry; it gets easier with time. She'll have less equipment attached, and you'll get to be a pro at dealing with dangling wires.

Knowing what to expect with a premature baby

Premature babies don't exactly look like the babies you have pictured in your mind, especially if they weigh less than 5 pounds (2.2kg). If your baby is born before 35 weeks, this is what she may look like:

- ✔ **Skinny:** Babies born before 35 weeks often don't have a good layer of fat.

- ✔ **Big-eyed:** The lack of fat in her face gives your prem baby a wide-eyed look.

- ✔ **Thin-skinned:** The blood vessels are more visible in a prem baby's skin.

- ✔ **Hairy – except on her head:** Prem babies are often still covered with *lanugo*, fine downy hair that helps keep them warm before they develop enough subcutaneous (under-the-skin) fat. Babies born before 26 weeks, on the other hand, may have no hair anywhere, and may have very red, gelatinous- looking skin.

- ✔ **Boys may have underdeveloped genitalia:** Don't worry, dad – they'll grow.

If you think the baby looks really odd, check with the nurses for reassurance that everything's okay, but not within your partner's earshot. No matter what she looks like, your partner is going to think she's the most beautiful person on the planet.

 Parents often have a sixth sense or are just more observant of the little changes in their babies and may notice a change in their condition before the staff does. Don't be afraid to speak up if you feel something's not right!

Clarifying common problems

Premature babies often have respiratory problems because their lungs aren't well developed. Artificial ventilation may be started almost immediately and will gradually be decreased as the baby tolerates the decrease in extra oxygen. Some babies need special types of ventilation to overcome resistance in their lungs.

Most premature babies have feeding problems. Tiny babies, under 28 weeks, may not be fed by mouth for weeks or months, because their digestive systems are too immature to handle food. Intravenous feeding is given instead and, as the baby grows, tube feeding is started. Feeding the baby through a nipple on a bottle is begun very slowly, because sucking can tire a prem baby and use up her energy stores.

Many babies grow very slowly in the NICU. Infections, stress and any number of complications can slow growth. Reading the weight chart and seeing the weight increase by a few grams can be the highlight of a NICU parent's day.

Learning the ropes (and wires!)

Sometimes knowing what's what when it comes to the wires and machines attached to your baby can calm your anxiety. Your average prem baby may sport the following wires and attachments:

Breathing apparatus

If the baby can't breathe on her own, she may be attached to a ventilator via a tube that goes through her mouth or nose down to her lungs. This delivers a certain number of breaths per minute. Alternatively, she may be attached to nasal prongs, which deliver extra oxygen to her lungs via – naturally – prongs that fit into her nose. Try very hard not to do anything that may dislodge the breathing tubes.

Monitoring equipment

Since prem babies have an unfortunate habit of forgetting to breathe, often even babies who don't need breathing equipment are hooked up to a monitor that flashes a series of incomprehensible numbers, some with little flashing hearts next to them. The monitor is attached to the baby by wires that lead from her chest, and possibly also from her hand or foot, or even from her umbilical cord if a line was placed there right after birth.

The machines monitor pulse (that's the flashing heart), respiration, (the number of times the baby breathes each minute) and oxygenation levels. Prem babies' heart rates are from 110 to 160 beats per minute, on average. Respirations are 40 to 60 per minute. Oxygenation in the 90s is good. Blood pressure may also be continuously monitored in very sick babies.

The baby's temperature may also be monitored frequently, if not continuously. Because prem babies have little in the way of fat stores, they get cold easily, and stress and the extra work of being sick and trying to grow can use up energy that may otherwise help keep them warm. The incubator or bed the baby is laying on also has its own thermometer to make sure it doesn't get too hot or too cold.

Intravenous lines

Most NICU babies receive intravenous medications and nourishment, at least at first. IV lines can be very precarious in prem babies and need to be replaced frequently. The medications infused are sometimes hard on the veins, which 'blow', necessitating a new IV. The NICU nurses don't do it on purpose, believe us; spending time putting a new IV in a prem baby is rarely on the 'fun things to do in the NICU' list.

If your baby has an umbilical line, she may not have a peripheral line (a line in the extremities or head), but umbilical lines can't be used for very long because they're a potential source of infection.

Preparing for prem baby setbacks

Just when you think things are finally moving in the right direction, your premature baby may get sick. Because prem babies have decreased ability to fight off infection, and because they're attached to invasive equipment that can serve as a portal into the body, infections are very common. Some common NICU complications include the following:

- ✔ **Respiratory infection:** The tubes allow entry of germs into the lungs; pneumonia may develop and need antibiotic treatment.

- ✔ **Respiratory disease:** Long-term ventilation can save your baby's life but can also contribute to bronchopulmonary dysplasia – damage to the lungs that can take months or years to fully heal. This problem is more common in very tiny babies. Some babies with respiratory disease are discharged while still receiving oxygen, which is decreased gradually as they develop the ability to breathe better on their own.

- ✔ **Necrotising enterocolitis:** Called *NEC* by the NICU staff, this inflammation of the immature digestive system usually occurs after feeding is started. NEC can seriously damage the intestines. Feeds are temporarily stopped so the gut can heal, and IV feeds are given instead.

✔ **Intraventricular haemorrhage (IVH):** IVH is a bleed into the brain that can range from mild (graded I) to very serious (graded IV). Around a third of babies born between 24 and 26 weeks have a bleed, but any baby born before 34 weeks can have an IVH. Bleeds may occur at the time of delivery or afterward.

Taking baby home

Preterm babies don't always have to stay in the hospital until they reach their original due date, and they don't always have to weigh 5 pounds (2.2kg) before being discharged, either. NICUs generally assess the baby's condition, the parents' ability to handle possible problems and the parents' willingness to learn the baby's care so they can do it at home.

Many parents take home babies who are still being tube fed or who are on monitors to make sure they keep breathing. Others don't feel at all comfortable with technical equipment and would rather have their child in the hospital for a little longer to be monitored. In fact, feeling completely unprepared to take home a prem baby who has spent weeks or months in the NICU is very common.

If you or your partner starts to go into panic mode about home-coming, get involved with a premature baby support group (such as www.bliss.org.uk) if you haven't already. Knowing that other families have done this and the whole family has survived is very reassuring. And seeing a former 2-pounder racing around on her bike is the best possible assurance that most prem babies come through their early trauma just fine.

Seriously, going home with the inept pair of you is not the worst thing your baby will have to face in life, so just do it. Keep that NICU number on speed dial for a while, though!

Hi, Baby Baby Baby: Having Multiples

The birth rate of twins, triplets and more has exploded with the advent of in vitro fertilisation (IVF) and other advanced reproductive technology. Seventeen per cent of twins and 40 per cent of triplet births are results of infertility treatment. In 2009, out of 781,000 births in England and Wales, 12,595 were twins, 172 were triplets and 5 were quadruplets or more.

If you're expecting multiples, find a support group pronto. Not only are they a great source for used twin or triplet baby paraphernalia, which can be extremely expensive, but they're also a source of a lot of practical info on how to handle more than one baby.

Multiple identities: What multiples are and who has them

Although infertility treatments are the largest risk factor for multiples, you're more likely to have more than one baby if

- ✔ **Your partner is black.** Black women have the highest natural twinning rate of the different racial groups; Asian women have the lowest.

- ✔ **Your partner is older than 35.** Twins occur naturally around 3 per cent of the time in women aged 25 to 29, and 5 per cent of the time in women aged 35 to 39.

- ✔ **Fraternal twins (non-identical) run in her family.** Your family history doesn't seem to have any bearing on the statistics. If she's a fraternal twin, she has a 1 in 17 chance of having fraternal twins.

Twins can be either fraternal or identical. Fraternal twins are created from two different eggs and are no more similar than any other two siblings. Identical twins are the result of one embryo splitting into two at a very early stage of development. Siamese twins, also called conjoined twins, are always identical twins who didn't completely split as embryos. Conjoined twins are usually identified on ultrasound before delivery.

Obviously, boy–girl twins are always fraternal, but if you have two of the same sex, it may be difficult to tell at first whether they're identical or fraternal. The majority of twins, especially twins from IVF cycles, are fraternal, although IVF also increases the risk of having identical twins. DNA testing is the only definite way to determine if twins are identical or fraternal, although sometimes it's obvious twins are fraternal if they look quite different.

 Many IVF parents who implanted only two embryos have been surprised to find themselves carrying three foetuses. If this happens to you, don't accuse the doctor of putting in an extra embryo she had lying around! What happened was that one of the embryos split into identical twins.

Health risks for mum

All the usual pregnancy complaints are intensified during a multiple pregnancy. Annoying issues such as morning sickness, weight gain, heartburn, constipation, shortness of breath (especially on any type of exertion), urinary problems and haemorrhoids are all likely to be magnified.

Many of the health risks of pregnancy for your partner increase with the number of foetuses she's carrying. Multiple pregnancies are more often medically complicated by:

- **Gestational diabetes:** The increased placental size and hormone production may raise the risk of gestational diabetes in multiple pregnancies.

- **Pregnancy-induced hypertension:** High blood pressure after 20 weeks of pregnancy. One in three mothers of multiples develops PIH.

- **Anaemia:** Maternal low red blood cell count.

- **Haemorrhage:** Severe blood loss at the time of delivery.

- **Placental abruption:** Women with multiples are three times more likely to have the placenta come off the uterine wall prematurely, possibly resulting in severe haemorrhage.

- **Caesarean deliveries:** Caesarean deliveries are pretty much a given in high-order (triplets or more) multiple births because it's unlikely all the babies will be head down, and high-order multiples are so small that even if they're all head down before birth, one or more are very likely to flip as soon as the first baby is delivered and the rest have more room, possibly necessitating an emergency caesarean.

For high-order multiples, bed rest during pregnancy is very likely.

Risks for the babies

Twins are five times more likely than single babies to have problems at birth or to die before or soon after delivery. Multiple pregnancies often deliver early, since the uterus has less room for all the occupants, and preterm babies are known to have more complications, so these factors account for some but not all of the risks multiples face. Statistics show that

✔ Approximately 60 per cent of twins deliver before 37 weeks.

✔ Thirty-six per cent of triplets deliver before 32 weeks.

✔ Eighty per cent of quads and more deliver before 32 weeks.

Twins are also more likely to have the following complications:

✔ Twin-to-twin transfusion syndrome can occur only in identical twins who share the same placenta. One twin receives too much blood, the other too little. Both can cause problems.

✔ Birth defects such as cerebral palsy are much more common in multiples, and the risk increases with the number of foetuses.

✔ Cord accidents can occur, such as knots in the cord or entanglement in the cord. Cord accidents reduce blood flow to the foetus. Identical twins, who develop in one amniotic sac, are more likely to become entangled in their own or their twin's cord.

Your medical practitioner may well suggest that you deliver at a hospital equipped for high-risk births, but if they don't, you should still plan to do so. Knowing that your babies will have all the technological advances that may be needed in place from the moment of delivery can really reduce the stress you and your partner feel.

Chapter 7

In the Home Stretch: The Third Trimester

In This Chapter

▶ Seeing how baby gets ready for delivery in the third trimester

▶ Putting on weight and dealing with hormones: mum's last three months

▶ Maintaining some seclusion for you and your partner

*T*he last three months of pregnancy are when reality hits like a tonne of bricks and you and your partner realise, albeit still rather dimly, that a real baby is coming to live with you. A baby with his own personality; a separate person who is developing definite likes and dislikes even before birth and will be able to express them even when he can't say a word.

In the third trimester, all the major organs and appendages are in place, and all the baby has to do is grow. Mum is also doing her own growing, with an attendant list of common discomforts and complaints that you'll become well acquainted with. In this chapter we look at baby's growth, mum's growth and your part in dealing with your family's expansion.

Tracking Baby's Development during the Third Trimester

At the start of the third trimester, your baby is fully formed, although you wouldn't think so if you got a look inside the uterus. The eyes are still fused, the skin is gelatinous and the body fat is nonexistent, but everything that the baby needs to develop into a normal newborn is present and accounted for. The following sections provide the highlights of foetal development in the last three months of pregnancy.

Adding pounds and maturing in the seventh and eighth months

Week 27 starts off the final trimester of pregnancy, and don't think your partner will let you forget for one minute that she's been hauling this child around for six months already. While week 27 marks the beginning of the end of a full-term pregnancy, it also marks the end of the 'easy' trimester.

So if you thought you heard lots of complaints in months four, five and six, you ain't seen nothin' yet! And her complaints are justified. The baby grows from around 10in (25cm) long and 1.5lb (0.7kg) at week 27 to around 18in (46cm) long and 4 to 6lb (1.8 to 2.8kg) by week 36. That's a lot of growth in just nine weeks, and your partner will be feeling it.

In the seventh and eighth months, the baby develops in the following ways:

- ✔ **Fully develops the lung tissue necessary to breathe outside the uterus:** By 36 weeks, most babies can breathe independently without oxygen supplementation.

- ✔ **Matures the digestive tract and kidneys:** The ability to breathe, suck, swallow and eliminate in tandem is essential for life outside the uterus.

- ✔ **Begins to see:** The eyes open around week 31, and the baby begins to perceive light and darkness.

- ✔ **Jumps in response to loud noises and recognises familiar voices:** Go ahead, talk just to him – he'll turn toward your voice after he's born if he's familiar with it, and 'Darling, get me a beer' aren't the only sounds you want him to associate with you.

- ✔ **Puts on some fat:** Your baby gains weight in these nine weeks (and so does your partner) because the baby is both growing and developing fat stores to help him regulate his temperature after birth.

Figure 7-1 shows the development of your baby in these final weeks.

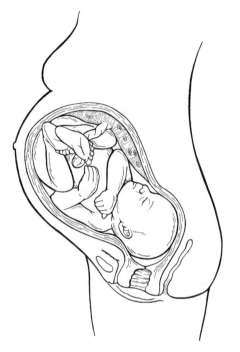

Figure 7-1: The foetus looks more and more like a fully developed person in the third trimester.

Getting everything in place in the ninth month

The ninth month is the home straight. In these four weeks the baby assumes the head-down position for good – at least you hope he does. After 36 weeks, he's usually too big to do somersaults, although some babies do manage to turn themselves right-side up, which, for birthing purposes, is upside down, or *breech*. (See Chapter 9 for more about breech deliveries.)

Your baby doesn't have much left to do in the last four weeks but grow and perfect already-in-place systems. In the last month, your baby will:

✔ **Have descended testicles, if he's a boy:** Earlier in pregnancy, the testicles develop in the abdomen and descend gradually into the groin before assuming their final position outside the body. Boys whose testicles don't descend by the time of birth are evaluated periodically. Surgery may be required if they don't descend by a certain age because the increased body temperature can damage reproductive organs in males.

✔ **Start to develop wake–sleep patterns:** Most babies seem to be more active at night, which may give you some idea of what you're in for.

✔ **Shed body hair and gain some head hair:** Lanugo, the soft downy hair that covers the foetus earlier in pregnancy, starts to disappear. Hair on the head may be abundant or nonexistent. Dark-skinned babies often have more hair at birth than future blondies.

✔ **Swallow amniotic fluid, urinate and practise breathing:** Babies get ready to eat by swallowing amniotic fluid, which also gives the kidneys practice in elimination as urine is excreted into the amniotic fluid.

✔ **Be active:** Some babies are thumb suckers even before birth. He may yawn, grimace and grab the umbilical cord in his hand. Kicking gets harder as space becomes tighter, and he's likely to stay in position – hopefully head down – without turning during the last month.

✔ **Drop lower into the pelvis:** In anticipation of labour, the baby may drop down so that his head is pressing more directly on the cervix. This pressure helps thin and dilate the cervix, and also helps prevent the umbilical cord from falling below his head if your partner's water breaks, a dangerous situation known as a cord prolapse. (See Chapter 9 for more about cord prolapse.)

Finding Out What Mum Goes Through in the Third Trimester

The baby isn't the only one who changes in these final months, of course. Although your partner's changes on the outside are obvious, if somewhat unnerving at times (Can she really get any bigger than this? Won't her skin break apart?), the changes on the inside are just as dramatic, if not more so.

Getting acquainted with your 'new' partner, now known as mother-to-be-with-a-vengeance, can be as complicated as getting to know the baby after he's born. Keep in mind at all times that she's going through physical and emotional upheavals the likes of which you'll never be able to fathom, but you need to try.

Understanding your partner's physical changes

A pregnant woman at the end of the second trimester still looks pretty much like her normal self. Your partner may not even be wearing maternity clothes at this point, letting large shirts (yours, probably) and trousers a size or two larger than her normal size cover her cute little belly. All that changes in the third trimester for most women, although some lucky women never look all that pregnant, even when delivering 8 pound (3.5kg) babies.

Between the seventh and ninth months, expect these changes in your partner's physique and physical condition:

- ✔ **The uterus can be felt** a few inches above her belly button at the start of the third trimester, and up under her ribs by the end.

- ✔ **Leg cramps** occur because of nerve compression by the growing uterus.

- ✔ **Backache** is common because of the strain from the additional weight in front.

- ✔ **Constipation and haemorrhoids** can occur as a result of sluggish, compressed bowels. Pain and rectal bleeding can accompany haemorrhoids. Stool softeners, drinking enough fluids and eating lots of roughage can help.

- ✔ **Urination** becomes almost a full-time job. She may need to get up in the night to urinate.

- ✔ **Varicose veins** may pop out on her legs; they may itch or ache. Spider veins, small broken capillaries, may also occur on her face, neck and arms.

- ✔ **Itchy skin** is a huge problem for some pregnant women in the third trimester. Creams help keep the skin moisturised and decrease itching.

- ✔ **Heartburn** becomes more severe, but despite old wives' tales, it's in no way related to the amount of hair the baby will have!

- ✔ **Feet and ankles often swell,** especially if you're having a summer baby. Encourage her to rest with her feet up as much as possible.

- ✔ **Her centre of gravity shifts,** making falls more likely. Hide her high heels and, if she'll let you, take her arm when walking, like a proper gentleman.

✔ **Shortness of breath comes with exertion,** because the baby is pressing on her lungs. When the baby drops, she may feel relief, but the tradeoff is increased frequency of urination.

✔ **She may have trouble sleeping,** even though she's always tired. Try tying a 6-pound (2.7-kg), baby-shaped weight to your abdomen and you'll quickly understand why.

✔ **Breasts may start leaking** a few drops of colostrum, the first fluids produced after birth. They may also look huge, since they contain around 2 pounds (1kg) of extra weight – each!

✔ **Vaginal discharge increases,** so expect the reappearance of panty liners in the bathroom cupboard.

✔ **Interest in sex** may be at either extreme; it may be the last thing she's interested in, or one of the things that interests her most. Hormones are funny that way. (See Chapter 4 for more about sex during pregnancy.)

Contractions may also begin to occur on and off, starting with Braxton Hicks contractions, which don't change the cervix and are felt mostly in the front of the abdomen rather than in the back.

As the due date approaches, more contractions may come and go, usually with just enough frequency to have you leaping for the suitcase and putting it in the car before they peter out. Don't worry; the real thing will start soon enough!

Heeding warning signs

Though many complaints of late pregnancy are normal and expected, some are not. Make sure your partner contacts her medical practitioner if she experiences any of the following symptoms:

✔ **Vaginal bleeding:** In the last few weeks of the pregnancy, her medical practitioner should be told about any type or amount of bleeding. Bleeding can indicate a placental detachment, called a placental abruption, or placenta praevia, a low-lying placenta. (See Chapter 6 for more about both conditions.) However, a *bloody show* (blood-tinged mucus) is a normal sign of impending labour and nothing to worry about.

✔ **A sudden severe headache:** Strong headaches can be a sign of pre-eclampsia. (See Chapter 6 for more on the risks of pre-eclampsia.)

✔ **Severe abdominal pain:** This can be a sign of placental abruption, the premature separation of the placenta from the uterine wall, which can be life threatening for mother and baby.

✔ **Swelling of her face, hands and feet:** Some swelling at the end of pregnancy is normal, but facial swelling can also be a sign of pre-eclampsia, especially if accompanied by sudden weight gain, headache or a rise in blood pressure.

✔ **Leaking fluid:** This symptom usually indicates the bag of waters has broken. This is normal at the end of pregnancy, but not in the seventh or eighth month. Always call if she notices more discharge than normal or is leaking fluid. After the water breaks, the baby is more susceptible to infection because its protective sac is breached. If labour doesn't begin within 24 hours, her medical practitioner may consider inducing labour.

Bracing yourself for your partner's emotional changes

Hormone levels are very high in the last few months of pregnancy, and, for many women, with hormones come mood swings. Be prepared for the following emotional changes in the last trimester:

✔ **Irritability:** When you don't feel your best physically, everything irritates you. Try not to be one of the 'everythings' that drives her crazy.

✔ **Weepiness:** Women find many reasons to cry in the last few months of pregnancy. They cry because they're happy, sad, frustrated or angry. They cry for reasons they can't even express to you, which can, of course, be frustrating for you, but you'll get over it.

✔ **Self-image issues:** Pregnancy changes a woman's body image, sometimes for the better, sometimes not. Some women resent the loss of the perfect figure, while others are happy that pregnancy provides an excuse for the extra weight that's always bugged them. Expect to hear her make negative comments, and don't respond to them in kind. The answer to 'Do I look fat?' is never 'Yes'.

Some degree of moodiness, sadness or depression is normal, but mood changes in late pregnancy should be fleeting, not permanent. As many as 10 per cent of women become clinically depressed during pregnancy and need medical intervention, and up to 20 per cent develop some depressive symptoms that may also need medical treatment.

Pregnant dad symptoms: Couvade syndrome

In the past few years, some attention has been given to the idea that expectant dads may develop symptoms similar to those of their partners. Studies suggest that this phenomenon, known as *Couvade syndrome*, may affect as many as 90 per cent of dads-to-be. Weight gain, nausea, backache and other pregnancy symptoms may be experienced by dad as a psychological or physical reaction to his own weight gain, which may be the result of eating more from stress or just from keeping up with his partner. Whatever the reason, rest assured in the third trimester that if you have 'pregnancy pains', they too will soon be coming to an end.

Symptoms of clinical depression include sadness that doesn't lift, feelings of hopelessness or guilt, difficulty sleeping, constant fatigue or behaviour not typical for her. Don't ignore depression that seems extreme or that doesn't lift after a few days. (See Chapter 12 for more on depression after pregnancy.)

Antidepressant medications can be given in pregnancy if your partner's medical practitioner feels the benefits outweigh the risks – certain antidepressants known as *selective serotonin re-uptake inhibitors* may increase the risk of heart defects, respiratory problems, low muscle tone, irritability and eating difficulties in the newborn. In 2010 the MHRA's Drug Safety Update included a review of epidemiological data suggesting that use of selective serotonin reuptake inhibitors (SSRIs) in pregnancy, particularly in the later stages, may increase the risk of persistent pulmonary hypertension in the newborn (PPHN). The observed risk was approximately 5 per 1,000 pregnancies vs. background rate in general population of 1 to 2 per 1,000 pregnancies.

Sympathising with her desire to get this over with

Around the seventh month, many women start expressing a strong desire to have this pregnancy over and done with. Before you jump in with long-winded explanations of how the baby isn't fully developed yet, it's too early and other pompous statements about why being pregnant for just two more months is a good idea, realise that she isn't really wanting to have the baby early (well, maybe she is, a little); she's just tired and frustrated with being pregnant.

The last few months of pregnancy are no picnic, and unfortunately, you can't truly understand what she's going through. When she starts talking about getting this baby out by hook or by crook the minute she hits 37 weeks, take it with a pinch of salt. She's every bit as concerned about the welfare of this baby as you are, and she's not going to do anything rash.

Let her vent without giving her a lecture, and in five minutes she'll probably be telling her mum how pregnancy has been the best time of her life. That's how hormones go sometimes.

Dealing with tears, panic and doubts

Doing anything for the first time can be stressful, overwhelming and scary. Facing labour, delivery and motherhood for the first time certainly qualifies. Yes, you're also facing fatherhood for the first time, and dealing with the prospect of labour, seeing your partner in pain and a host of doubts and fears, but her concerns are fuelled by hormones and the knowledge that some form of delivery, be it labour or surgery, is the only way to emerge with a baby after nine months of pregnancy. The inevitability of the end of pregnancy can be overwhelming at times.

Your partner won't be the first woman to ever express the feeling that she can't do this, that having a baby was a mistake or that she's changed her mind about the whole thing and wants to call it off. These feelings will intensify when she's in labour, so if you deal with them rationally now, you'll be better prepared for them then.

These feelings are temporary, but they're overwhelming when they hit. All new parents fear they won't be good at their new role. The two of you can approach this fear together by taking the following practical steps:

- ✔ **Read baby books and check out websites.** You'll still go to pieces during the first colic episode, but if you know what to expect, it's a little easier to handle.

- ✔ **Take a class.** Most hospitals offer pregnancy classes that touch on at least the basics of breastfeeding and newborn care.

- ✔ **Visit friends with babies.** If you have friends or relatives with infants, hang out with them and pick their brains, if you trust their judgement.

✔ **Talk to your mum and dad.** Although time dims the memories of parenting, your own parents may be able to vaguely recall their early parenting days and give you some advice based on their own experiences. After all, you turned out okay, didn't you? If you didn't, don't ask them.

✔ **Talk it out.** Experience may change your mind about a number of parenting issues, but you'll feel more prepared if the two of you try to set out some basic ideas about how you want to raise the baby. Chewing over a few things now helps avoid drama-filled discussions when one of you wants to put the baby in your bed at 3 a.m. and the other doesn't, and also gives you the sense of having some grasp of what parenthood is all about. Expect your ideas to change frequently in the first actual weeks of parenthood, though.

Allow your partner to vent and express doubts and concerns, but never fail to reassure her that you know she'll be a great mum, that she was born to do this and that you'll be helping her every inch of the way. Feel free to express your own fears and doubts about being a really good parent, but never in a 'Can you top this' way.

Many women at the end of pregnancy have very vivid dreams about the baby or develop fears that something may be wrong with him. You can't do much about these fears except let her talk them out and reassure her that no matter what happens, you're there for her and the baby. However, if your partner becomes fixated on thoughts that she may harm the baby or that something is wrong with the baby, she may be experiencing a severe depressive disorder. Make sure she sees her medical practitioner promptly.

Facing your own fears about fatherhood

Today's new dads may not have had involved fathers as role models as they were growing up, which can lead to uncertainty about exactly how to approach fatherhood. The idea that dad should be as involved in child rearing as mum is a fairly new one, and you may feel uncertain about your role.

Because no two families are alike, you and your partner will design your own family model. You set your own standards here, so don't worry about what a 'good' dad does or how other people approach fatherhood. You're going to be a 'good' dad, so however you decide to embrace the parenting role will be the right thing for you and your partner.

Whose Baby Is This, Anyway? Dealing with Overbearing Family Members

From the time you share the news of your coming baby, you'll be inundated with advice and visitors. Nobody will want to be more hands-on than your family, and it may grow tiresome and become a source of angst very quickly the closer to labour and delivery your partner gets, and especially when you get home from the hospital and crave some family time.

Mothers, grandfathers, aunts-to-be – they all get nervous, too. Unfortunately, their offers of assistance and their constant presence can keep you and your partner from some much-needed quiet bonding time before baby arrives. Your lives are about to change forever, for the better (baby, baby, baby!) and for the worse (goodbye sleep and frequent sex!), and you need time to enjoy the waning bits of childlessness you have left.

Your families love you, and their well-meaning, obtrusive advice, visits and purchases are the only way they know how to show you just how excited they are to meet the new little person you're bringing into the family. However, if members of your family are becoming too involved or over-the-top for your taste, be sure to thank them for the love and support and simply let them know that you and your partner need to take some time for yourselves before the baby comes.

Depending on how big and how emotionally connected your family is, consider starting a phone tree to share news earlier in your pregnancy to save you from having to call every single relative in your phone book every time you go in for an ultrasound (see Chapter 8 for details on creating a phone tree). Telling the same story over and over to 13 aunts, cousins and neighbours may take the fun right out of your fun news. That said, don't cut off communication altogether. Make sure to call the most important people in your life as frequently as you see fit. It's an exciting time for everyone, and you won't want to tarnish a loved one's joy by letting him get all the news second hand.

Chapter 8

The Co-Pilot's Guide to Birthing Options

· ·

· ·

*L*abour is nothing like it used to be. From the au naturel days when biting down on a bullet was the 'medication' and the 1950s when every woman was sedated up to her eyeballs while dad spent the night in the pub, labour has evolved into a family event that involves medications that really take the pain out of labour, sleepovers for dad and champagne dinners the night before discharge.

One thing about having a baby is sure: there's no one right way to do it. For every person who wants to deliver at home on her grandma's favourite quilt, another person feels that *epidural on demand* is the best phrase in the English language. Whatever you and your partner dream up as the ideal labour experience, rest assured it probably won't be the weirdest idea your doctor or midwife has ever heard.

You have more childbirth options today than ever before. Natural deliveries, home deliveries and give-me-everything-you've-got deliveries are all possible. And the good thing is, no one is going to hold your partner to the ideas you both thought sounded good before labour started. If she decides she wants an epidural after all, all she has to do is say so (believe us, you'll hear her!).

Although the number of options is much larger than in previous years, some of them may not be feasible in your situation. For instance, if your partner has certain medical conditions, such as pre-eclampsia, or if the baby has congenital birth defects, they really need to be under a doctor's care in a hospital, even if your partner had her heart set on a home delivery. Be sure to talk to the doctor early in the pregnancy about your plans so that she can advise you on their feasibility and safety and let you know if circumstances change.

In this chapter we review the options that are available and help you decide what works best for you and your partner. We also provide tips on crafting a birth plan and deciding who's allowed in the delivery room.

Make sure you and your partner are agreed on what you want before discussing plans with your medical practitioners, and discuss it well before labour starts. Arguing in front of the nurses and trying to talk your partner out of having an epidural at 6 centimetres dilation is considered really bad form by the hospital staff, and they may not let you use the coffee machine or show you their hidden stash of emergency snacks for fainting fathers if they don't like the way you talk to your partner!

Choosing Where to Deliver

A century ago, everyone delivered at home. Fifty years ago, everyone delivered in the hospital. Today parents can choose either option, or may deliver in a special birthing centre designed to mimic the comforts at home while still providing cutting-edge medical treatment if needed.

Delivering at a hospital

Hospitals today love to stress how much like home they are while still having all the most up-to-date equipment at their fingertips. But, although hospitals have come a long way in improving the overall birthing experience, they're still not home. Some, however, are better than others at creating a welcoming, open-door policy for family, so check out your local hospital. Here's what to look for:

✔ **Is it secure?** Most hospitals have beefed up security, especially around the maternal and child health area. Hospital bracelets embedded with alarm triggers are sometimes available, codes have to be activated to enter certain areas and the staff all dress in one colour so you know who belongs there. It should *not* be possible to just walk onto a maternity floor without a pass. You want security to be tight, even if it's a pain in the neck.

✔ **What visiting policies exist?** What you're looking for depends on your preferences. Do you want your entire family and a three-piece band present, or are you hoping to have just the two of you at the delivery and in the maternity ward afterward? Keeping family out is much easier if you can quote 'hospital rules'.

✔ **How much access does dad have?** Many places allow dad 24-hour visiting privileges, but some don't. Find out the rules ahead of time so security isn't called to remove you.

✔ **Are the staff helpful?** You can tell a lot by the attitude of the staff, even on a short visit. Do they smile and say hello, or run over your foot with a trolley without even an 'excuse me'? Although you may still draw a tired or stressed midwife, it's less likely at a hospital with a mission statement and policies that promote a positive atmosphere.

✔ **Is anaesthesia available all night?** Surprising as it may be, some small hospitals don't have an anaesthetist in the hospital all night. The anaesthetist may have to be called in from home if your partner wants an epidural during the night. And if the hospital has only one on staff, she may be starting another operation just as your partner starts getting really uncomfortable. Know ahead of time so you can ask for an epidural early, if need be.

✔ **How's the décor?** Consider the appearance of the hospital room after everything else has been taken into consideration. Pretty surroundings are nice, but you'll be too busy to notice them.

After you make your decision, visit the hospital again if you can. Knowing exactly what the ward looks like and even recognising some familiar faces removes a layer of stress as you get ready for delivery. Some hospitals offer tours so ask if this option is available to you.

While you're there, take note of the eating options, parking guidelines and classes offered by the hospital. This information allows you to plan ahead and offer your well-wishers the information they need as well as the opportunity to make full use of the facility's offerings.

Some hospitals offer breastfeeding classes run by specialist nurses. Post-delivery, these nurses can then visit women who are struggling with breastfeeding. Encourage your partner to attend a class in order to learn the basics of breastfeeding as well as to initiate a face-to-face relationship with the specialist nurse who runs it. Your partner will be much more comfortable asking questions and discussing any issues she and baby are having if she has met the specialist previously.

Exploring alternative options: Using a midwife at home

The idea of having your baby at home may appeal to you and your partner. Home delivery may be an option for you if you meet all the following strongly suggested guidelines:

✔ You live fairly close to a hospital in case of emergencies.

✔ You're not delivering in John O'Groats in January or any other area where roads are impassable during the part of year you're due.

✔ You're both calm, sensible people who are really committed to the idea of home birth.

The trouble with labour is that while 99 out of 100 times everything goes perfectly, you need to be prepared for that one time when things go bad so quickly you can't believe your eyes. Having nearby medical help is really essential, unless your midwife can do a caesarean in under 30 minutes in an emergency!

Discuss with your GP circumstances that may cause you to change your mind about home delivery, from ominous weather to last-minute cold feet.

If you plan to use a midwife at home, be sure to get good answers to the following questions:

✔ **What type of equipment will you bring with you?** You can be sure a ventilator and fully equipped operating room won't appear out of her black bag, but basic medications like intravenous fluids and medication to prevent heavy bleeding after delivery and oxygen, plus equipment like an ambu bag to breathe for the baby in case of problems after birth, should be in every midwife's bag.

✔ **How long do you stay?** 'As long as you need me' is a good answer. She should stay at least an hour or two to make sure your partner and the baby are behaving normally and to get breastfeeding started. On the other hand, you may not want her moving in with you – that's your mother-in-law's role. She should also visit for the next few days to check both mother and baby in case of any late-developing problems.

Looking at Labour Choices

Standard labour practices vary depending on who is delivering and where you deliver, but no matter the situation, you and your partner will have to make a number of decisions and can opt to make dozens of others if you have preferences. Educate yourselves on common procedures and their pros and cons by talking with the doctor and doing some reading. One of the biggest issues for women in labour is deciding whether or not to have an epidural or other pain medication. In this section we discuss that as well as another big issue, water births.

Going all natural or getting the epidural

The decision about pain medication is one area where, although you're welcome to have your say – if you say it nicely – the decision is really up to your partner. As long as she's not planning to do anything unsafe, she's the one who has to go through labour, not you, so the drug decision should be hers.

The *all-natural* method of childbirth, which avoids unnecessary pain medication and medical interventions such as *episiotomies* (an incision on the perineum to make the vaginal opening larger), seems to have peaked about the time the hippie movement went mainstream and started buying BMWs, but letting nature take its course in childbirth still has many proponents. Women have been having babies naturally since forever, and many women find going through labour without any medication empowering.

Classes that teach breathing and relaxation techniques as a natural way to deal with pain are available. Some classes focus on specific breathing patterns, while others stress learning to listen to your body, relaxation methods and the benefits of staying upright during labour.

Around 50 per cent of women in labour these days have *epidurals*, an injection that numbs the nerves from the abdomen down to the thighs. Epidurals are usually given when labour is well established, around 4 centimetres dilation, because contractions can slow down if it's given too early. Some doctors, though, order epidurals earlier and then start a labour-inducing drug if contractions slow down.

Epidurals are better than they used to be; they can be run as a continuous infusion on a pump so they don't wear off and need to be re-injected. Some hospitals offer 'walking epidurals', where the dose given still allows patients to walk, which is better for keeping labour going than lying in bed.

Some women turn down the epidural but are given intravenous pain medications to help with labour pains. One problem with IV medications is that they can depress the baby's ability to breathe after birth, so they can't be given too close to the time of delivery.

Taking it to the water

Water birth is delivery of the baby while the mother is in a large tub of water. The baby is delivered while under the water, which is considered by proponents of the practice to be less traumatic to her because she's spent nine months in water. Although water birth sounds like a warm, back-to-nature experience, no cultures actually practise water birth. This fact doesn't mean that water birth doesn't have some appealing possibilities, mostly for mum-to-be, who gets to spend most of her labour floating in a tub of water. Many women find spending some time in labour in water reduces pain and aids in relaxation.

Babies have never been traditionally born into a vat of water, and although most babies don't breathe until they're out of the water, a few baby deaths have been related to water birth. Labouring in water and getting out for the actual delivery may be a safer option to consider.

Some women absolutely should not have a water birth. The list includes:

- ✔ Women giving birth prematurely. (See Chapter 6 for more on preterm delivery.)

- ✔ Women with genital herpes.

- ✔ Women whose babies have passed *meconium*, the first stool, before delivery. These babies need their mouth and nose suctioned as soon as the head is delivered, to help prevent meconium aspiration into the lungs.

Creating a Birth Plan

A birth plan is a document that outlines the procedures, medications and contingency plans that you and your partner are comfortable with throughout labour and delivery. It details your ideal birth experience while acknowledging the unpredictability of the process.

A birth plan is not a set of marching orders for your midwife or doctor, so keep it simple and friendly. You share this document with your entire birthing team, and not all doctors and midwives are thrilled at the prospect of a couple telling them how to do their jobs.

Creating a birth plan requires that you and your partner discuss what you're comfortable with and make many important decisions prior to your arrival at the hospital. The last thing you want to do is to leave life-altering, labour-changing decisions to be made during an emotionally wrought time.

Visualising your ideal experience

Labour and delivery are like reading a choose-your-own-adventure novel; every decision you make can lead you to a slightly different outcome.

As corny as it may sound, you and your partner should spend some time with your eyes closed trying to picture what your perfect experience would look like. Try to be realistic – a pain-free, 60-minute labour is highly unlikely, and making that dream a reality is beyond your control. Instead, focus on the things you can control.

When creating a birth plan, consider the following basic questions:

- ✔ What types of medication is your partner willing/wanting to have administered?
- ✔ Do you want to cut the umbilical cord?
- ✔ Does your partner want final approval before the doctor performs a vacuum extraction? This involves a suction device that helps pull the baby out, which can cause painful tearing of the vagina as well as temporarily misshapen baby heads.

> It is a safe and, in some cases, necessary procedure, but many women want to have the choice as to whether or not it is performed.

✔ Does your partner want constant or intermittent foetal monitoring? Foetal monitoring tracks baby's stress levels during childbirth, and constant monitoring will limit your partner's ability to move freely during labour.

✔ Does your partner want to veto an episiotomy? An episiotomy is a surgical incision that enlarges the vaginal opening to allow the baby to come out more easily. It used to be a common procedure, but most studies show that letting the body tear naturally is a better option. An episiotomy is quite painful during recovery and not an attractive option for most women unless absolutely necessary for the health of the baby.

✔ Does your partner want to be able to get up and walk around while labouring?

In order to make sure you both feel positive about your childbirth experience, you need to prepare answers to these important questions. Many procedures may be done as a matter of course that might not sit comfortably with your and your partner's desires, so invest the time beforehand in order to avoid any regrets regarding incidents that you could have prevented.

Many prenatal classes include exercises that help you visualise your ideal experience, and some even offer help developing your birth plan. When selecting a class, ask the instructor if these activities are included as part of the course. Having a third party involved may help you and your partner narrow down your list of what's truly important and turn those priorities into a cohesive, effective birth plan.

Drafting your plan

After you and your partner have decided what your ideal birth looks like, you need to put it into writing. Try to use language that's friendly, concise and represents your willingness to be flexible.

Births don't usually go exactly according to plan, so allow wiggle room for the unexpected to make sure the midwives and doctors know that your priority is having a healthy baby at the end of the day. Here are some basic tips for writing your birth plan:

✔ Write a nice, short introduction that introduces who you are and thanks your team in advance for following your plan.

✔ Include a brief overview that states your basic, overall desires for the kind of labour and delivery you and your partner want.

✔ Break the main body into three sections: labour, delivery and post-delivery.

✔ Under each heading, make the major points into a bulleted list for easy reading.

Keep your birth plan to one page unless you know ahead of time that your labour and delivery are going to be complicated and therefore require more steps.

Since the majority of what's being outlined in the birth plan is up to your partner to decide and ultimately undergo, get involved in this project by taking the lead. Make her favourite dinner and start a dialogue. Ask her questions about what she wants and tell her what you want, too. Take notes during your discussion and then start composing your birth plan. It won't happen overnight, but it will let her know how involved you want to be.

Use the following birth plan as an outline for creating an effective, concise document for your team:

The Johnson Birth Plan

The Midwives at City General Hospital

Parents: Rachel & Evan Johnson

We're looking forward to having our baby at City General Hospital with the midwives and staff! We know you see a lot of birth plans and we thank you for reading ours.

We anticipate a normal birth and would like to allow the process to unfold naturally. However, in the unlikely event of a complication, we will co-operate fully after an informed discussion with the birth team has taken place. We are also willing to sign release forms if legally required in order to avoid 'routine' procedures we opt against.

Overall, we would like no medication, examination or procedure to be administered to mother or baby until it is explained to us and we have given our consent. Thank you in advance for all of your hard work and excellent care!

Labour:

> ✔ *I would like to attempt labour without pain medication – I will ask (loudly, I'm sure!) if I feel I need something.*
>
> ✔ *We prefer intermittent, external foetal monitoring to continuous or internal. We consent to admission strip monitoring.*

Delivery:

> ✔ *I would like to have freedom of movement and position during delivery – squatting, hands and knees, and so on.*
>
> ✔ *I very strongly prefer natural tearing to an episiotomy.*
>
> ✔ *We very strongly prefer delaying cord cutting until the cord has stopped pulsating (consent for exception will be considered if baby is in distress or excess meconium is present).*
>
> ✔ *If surgery is required, Evan needs to be present. I prefer regional anaesthesia rather than general, except in case of an emergency.*

Post-delivery:

> ✔ *Please place baby on mother's abdomen immediately. We would like the baby to remain with parents at all times.*
>
> ✔ *We would like to start breastfeeding as soon as possible and delay potential interruptions.*

Thank you for your sensitivity to our preferences and for bringing your knowledge and care to this great event in our lives.

As important as this day is, you are not a celebrity, and your unrealistic demands won't be met with a smile and a nod. Nor will your team take any unnecessary risks that could harm mother or baby just to meet the requirements of your birth plan. Keep your birth plan focused on the elements of the birthing process that can be controlled, take each hurdle one at a time and, if and when things begin to deviate from the plan, help your partner to make the best decisions possible by getting detailed information about the risks and benefits from the knowledgeable members of your team.

Sharing your birth plan with the world

Unfortunately, labour usually doesn't begin on that imprecise due date you've been hanging your hat on for the last nine months.

Babies can come early, and with so much to get ready for, you may find yourself putting off creating and sharing your birth plan. Make time to write your birth plan toward the beginning of the third trimester, which will give you plenty of time to share it with your birthing team and any inquiring relatives and friends.

Going over your plan with the birthing team

Have your birth plan in place far in advance of your due date so that you can share it with your doctor and midwife during the seventh or eighth month of pregnancy. That gives you time to discuss the plan and address any concerns either may have.

Upon arrival at your delivery room, give a copy of your birth plan to the midwife assigned to your room. Hang a copy on the front of your door if permitted, as well as on the wall in your room, preferably near where your partner will deliver.

Informing family and friends of your plan

Conveying your plans early and often is key to getting everyone on the same page – or at least reading the same book – by the time the big day rolls around. Even if you can't get everyone to agree with your decisions, don't sweat it. Thank everyone for their concerns, but assure them that you would never make a decision that wasn't both educated and in the best interest of your partner and child. And, at the end of the day, when the baby arrives nobody will care how she got here.

Unless you're openly soliciting advice from others in your lives, talk about the plan as if it were a done deal. Talking about considerations and decisions you're making with a larger group of people means that, although you may get a wide spectrum of opinions, you'll also get an even wider spectrum of criticism when your decision doesn't adhere to everyone else's recommendations. However, you and your spouse have the right to decide the birthing option that works best for you. When your plan is in place, simply tell the people in your lives where, when and how you plan on having the baby.

If you and your partner are worried about the reaction your mother-in-law will have to the news of your plans to have an at-home water birth, don't be afraid to share the news of your personal birth plan via email. That way she's allowed to have her reaction without making you feel judged. Also, the more unconventional your birth plan is, the more information your family and friends will want about your choices. In those instances, it is best to formulate a detailed, concrete birth plan before sharing the information.

Many people are quite opinionated when it comes to whether or not to have a medicated labour. Don't feel the need to argue your position; the decision is ultimately yours, and what you want most is to do what's best for mother and baby in your eyes. Consider telling people that you plan on seeing how the events unfold and that you'll address mum's and baby's needs as you see fit on delivery day. After all, nobody knows what your partner will need or want until she's actually in labour.

Educate yourself on your options and be honest with your friends and family. If all else fails and someone still insists you're wrong, have a confrontation. Arguments aren't enjoyable, but you'll be happier if you have it hashed out before the big day arrives.

Picking the Cast: Who's Present, Who Visits and Who Gets a Call

Labour and delivery aren't the times for a family reunion. Having a baby is exhausting, emotional and the one time in your lives when you need to focus on each other and your baby more than anything else in the world. Which means that you and your partner probably won't want many people in the room with you. To avoid any arguments or awkwardness at the hospital when you should be focusing on other matters, decide in advance who you'll allow in the room for delivery, who can visit at the hospital and how you're going to spread news of the birth to everyone who isn't present.

Deciding who gets to attend the birth

Deciding who gets to be in the room is a big decision that's not yours to make. Your partner's the one nearly naked under a spotlight in a room of people, so she gets to make the call on who is allowed to be in the room during labour and delivery. And gentlemen, let's face it – she just may not want your mother there, no matter how much your mother would like to be present. As labour progresses, most women won't care who sees what because they'll be so focused on birthing the baby, but it's still best for her labour to have only the people she wants to have present. Any stress or distraction in early labour can slow down the process.

In addition to you, the midwife or doctor, some women opt to have a sister or close friend in the room who can provide her with much-needed emotional support. Other women decide to have one or both parents present. Again, check with your hospital to see who (and how many) they allow to be present for a birth.

Telling family members or friends that they need to leave isn't easy, but if your partner doesn't want someone in the room, it's your job to politely ask him or her to exit. For instance, if her father won't stop offering unsolicited stories about how painful his foot surgery was in comparison to her labour and she's on the verge of clobbering him with forceps, pull him aside, thank him for being there to support you both, let him know that your partner sends her love and then firmly explain that she's feeling the need to have silence in the room for the remainder of the delivery.

Of course this message won't go down well, but it's not about other people at this point. Put your partner's needs first and worry about hurt feelings later. Besides, the moment baby arrives, nobody will remember anything other than how perfect and amazing your new bundle of joy is.

Planning ahead for visitors

Many people opt to have no friends or family members present in the delivery room. But it also goes beyond that. Being inundated with visitors at the hospital may seem like a nice thing in theory, but in practice it can become overwhelming very quickly. You'll be tired, and your partner and baby will need rest, so make sure to take enough time for yourselves.

Also, having too many people handle your newborn only increases the risk of spreading illness. Invite only the most important people in your lives to the hospital and save the rest for a home visit in the following weeks. Thank anyone who offers to come and tell them that you look forward to spending time with them in the coming weeks. Simply telling someone that your new family will need rest, not visitors, should do the trick.

However, if someone shows up unannounced who you'd rather not have at the hospital, don't be afraid to tell her that you have to keep visits short, say five minutes or so, because your partner and baby need time to rest. Schedule a follow-up visit if you wish. If there's someone who you don't want allowed into your room, for safety reasons or otherwise, be sure to alert the staff of the person's name and description.

There's never been a better time in your life to focus inward, so don't spend time worrying about what other people will think about your decisions. You can always make up later if someone is offended.

Planting a phone tree

Spreading the news far and wide can be both exhausting and time consuming, and after a delivery you and your partner likely won't be up for talking to everyone you know. Nor will you have the time! Nonetheless, everyone you know will ask to be alerted within seconds after baby's arrival in the world.

Here are some simple tips to make a phone tree, which will require you to make only one call in order for the news of baby's arrival to begin branching out into the world.

1. **Start by gathering all the names and phone numbers of people you want contacted after your baby is born.**

2. **Start a list, with the first person as your primary contact.** He or she will be the one person you call upon baby's arrival.

3. **Write two names side-by-side under the primary contact.** These are the people your primary contact will call.

4. **Branching off those two people, write two more names under each.** The two people your primary contact calls will each have these two phone calls to make. Continue making the phone tree, assigning each person two calls.

5. **Pass out copies of the phone tree to everyone on the list and instruct them that when they get the call, they're responsible for calling the next two people straight away.**

   The phone tree still works if your callers have to leave phone messages, but the delay will slow down the rest of the communication.

If your list of contacts is short, consider having each person call just one other person.

Social network announcements

Sending an update to 500 of your nearest and not-so-nearest friends every time you have a witty musing about your favourite celebrity may be fun on the average day, but it may not be appropriate during labour and delivery.

Your partner may want you to keep the world abreast of the baby developments while she's in labour, but most women will prefer that your focus be on soothing her and not navigating your mobile phone.

A word of warning: as easy as it is to communicate using social networking sites, sharing major news, such as the birth of your child, via Facebook or Twitter will be offensive and hurtful to some of the more important people in your life. Finding out your best friend's baby arrived via a status update that already has 75 comments will leave those who truly love you feeling a bit cold. Take their feelings into consideration when making announcements throughout the pregnancy process. Make sure to hold off any major announcements until your phone tree has been initiated.

However, after news of the baby has spread through the appropriate channels to the appropriate people, social networking sites are a great way to show off your new bundle of joy to the adoring masses. It may cut down on the number of visits and phone calls you'll receive when you're basking in the glow of new fatherhood.

Part III
Game Time! Labour, Delivery and Baby's Homecoming

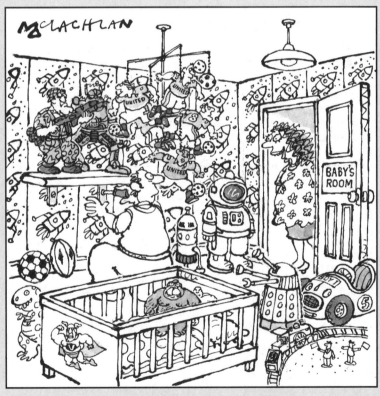

*"The hospital made a mistake with my scan—
It's a girl!"*

In this part...

If you want to be prepared for labour and delivery as well as the first hectic days at home, this part gives you all the necessary details. From knowing what to do when labour starts to feeding concerns and understanding the contents of the baby's nappy, the chapters in this part equip you to handle the big and little events and changes that take place in all your lives in a very short time span.

Chapter 9

Surviving Labour and Delivery

- -

In This Chapter

▶ Determining when labour is really happening

▶ Providing the best support possible

▶ Understanding the normal physical and medical aspects of labour

▶ Dealing with labour pain

▶ Needing a caesarean section

- -

*N*o matter how many birth plans you write (refer to Chapter 8 for more on writing a birth plan), and how many times you suffer through your relatives' birth stories, labour always comes as a surprise. For many guys, it's the first time you see your partner in real pain. Even worse, you know it's your fault – because she reminds you of that fact every five minutes. The end result will be worth it, though, so fasten your seat belt and get ready for the roller-coaster ride of labour and delivery.

No two labours are alike, so we can't say exactly what will happen in your partner's labour. The only thing most labours have in common is a beginning and an end, and still, labour can begin in a number of ways and can end in an operating theatre, hospital delivery suite, back seat of the car (not to scare you) or in your own bedroom. Although details differ, knowing approximately how labour will go can reduce your anxiety by, well, maybe a little bit.

When It's Time, It's Time – Is It Time?

Although you may think you won't have trouble telling when your partner is in labour, you may. Contractions often get closer as labour progresses, but sometimes they don't. Some women are in a lot of pain in labour, and some aren't.

All this confusion over the start of labour may have you leaping into the car every time your partner sighs during the last month of pregnancy; an actual moan may have you reaching for the phone to call 999. Take 999 off your speed dial, though; labour isn't always clear cut, but you can follow a few general rules when it comes to heading for the hospital:

- ✔ **If her waters break, call your medical practitioner (usually your midwife).** If you're having the baby in the hospital, your partner will be told to come in, even if she isn't having contractions. However, many women prefer to go through early labour at home, even after their waters break. Discuss this with your medical practitioner. After the waters break, your partner has an increased risk of infection and a small chance that the umbilical cord can *prolapse*, or fall below the baby's head.

- ✔ **If your partner's a Group B streptococcus carrier, go to the hospital as soon as her water breaks.** During pregnancy, some women test positive for Group B streptococcus, a common bacteria that can be carried in the vagina. The bacteria normally causes no harm in healthy women, but after the water breaks, beta strep can ascend up to the foetus and cause serious infection, so intravenous antibiotics usually need to be started right away. Not every woman has a vaginal swab specifically to check for group B streptococcal infection, but those that have a vagina swab for other reasons, during which it is picked up, are given antibiotics.

- ✔ **If your partner is in severe pain, even if the contractions are not regular, call your medical practitioner.** Pregnancy complications such as the placenta separating from the uterine wall, called *placental abruption*, can cause severe pain and can be life threatening.

- ✔ **If bleeding like a menstrual period occurs, call your medical practitioner.** A small amount of blood-tinged mucus is common when the mucus plug is passed, but heavier bleeding needs medical evaluation.

- ✔ **When contractions are regular and getting closer, call your labour ward.** They don't have to be – and may never be – five minutes apart.

Avoiding numerous dry runs (yes, it's us again)

Calling your midwife or doctor before going to the hospital and following their advice can save you many embarrassing excursions in and out of the labour and delivery ward. Think no one ever gets sent home without a baby? Think again. Think no one has ever been sent home ten or more times in a single pregnancy? Think again, again. And yes, the staff will remember you from last week, and the week before!

Many women have contractions in the last month of pregnancy. If your partner's contractions aren't becoming stronger or getting closer together, this probably isn't the real deal. Unless her waters break, she's in severe pain or she's bleeding, wait until contractions get stronger and closer together. Just being in the labour and delivery ward really doesn't speed up the birthing process.

Knowing when it's too late to go

When your partner can't walk or talk through contractions that are progressively stronger and closer together, it's really time to go to the hospital. You'll know this instinctively when she says, 'It's time to go *now*'. But if by some chance she's a woman with short labours and says she feels pressure, has to have a bowel movement or starts to push, dial 999, unless you personally want to deliver the baby on the back seat or hospital lawn. Most paramedics have delivered babies before, or at the very least have read the manual that tells them what to do.

If the paramedics don't arrive in time remember that rapid deliveries are usually uncomplicated, and your job may consist of calming your partner and not letting the baby fall on the floor.

In addition:

- ✔ **Don't pull on the cord or cut it.** Cutting the cord, dealing with the placenta and worrying about vaginal tears can be done by people more schooled in such things than you.

- ✔ **Dry the baby off and keep him warm.** Skin-to-skin contact with mum is ideal.

- ✔ **If the baby isn't breathing, flick his heels.** Don't slap him or turn him upside down, even if you've seen it in numerous films.

Don't dwell too much on the possibility of an unexpected home delivery. The odds are very small that a first labour will progress so quickly that the baby delivers at home.

Supporting Your Partner during Labour

Women in labour need lots of support. Your partner needs to hear that she's doing well, that things are progressing as they should and that she really can do this. Even if her mother, sister, and five of her dearest friends are with her, she needs *you*. Support means different things to different women, though, and your job is to figure out what she needs while in labour and do it.

Figuring out how she wants to be supported

Your partner may not be in a very talkative mood during labour, so asking her what she wants you to do may get you kicked right out of the room. This is one time in her life when she wants you to think for yourself and take action without being told what to do. Take the lead by offering choices. Ask her if she wants

- A back rub.
- A massage.
- A hand to hold.
- You to sit behind her and support her back.
- An epidural.
- You to kick her mum out of the room.
- Any of the other labour options you discussed before today.

Not taking the insults seriously

Women are not responsible for anything they say during labour, but you are, so don't get upset with any suggestions she makes about your anatomy or comments on your ancestry. (And she doesn't really mean what she said about your mother, either!)

Pain makes people say things they don't mean and may not even remember, so don't file away her remarks for another day. Vocalising the pain in this way is both healthy and normal.

Looking at What Happens during and after Labour

Although childbirth classes and books do their best to tell you what will happen in labour, the reality is very hard to describe. But since it's our job to give you all the facts you can handle, the following sections describe what the normal stages of labour look like.

First stage

The first stage of labour encompasses the time between the first labour pain and complete dilation, when your partner will begin to push. Because quite a few things happen during the first stage of labour, it's further broken down into early, active and transition stages of labour.

Early labour

Early labour is defined as the time between the start of labour and dilation of the cervix to 3 centimetres. This is the longest part of labour, sometimes lasting a day or two. During the early stage, contractions are often far apart and irregular. These early contractions thin and dilate the cervix. In late pregnancy, the cervix is thick, and the opening between the uterus and vagina is closed.

Normally the cervix thins before it begins to dilate, but no hard and fast rules exist. Many women are already somewhat thinned and dilated before labour begins.

Active labour

Things really start to move along during active labour, which is defined by regular contractions that become stronger and dilate the cervix from 4 to 10 centimetres. Active labour takes four to eight hours on average, although subsequent labours are often much shorter. A woman in active labour usually can't walk or talk through her contractions. She also may become a creature you haven't met before, one who knows words that may totally surprise you.

You need to be active in active labour, too. If your partner is attempting natural childbirth, she needs help staying focused and breathing through the contractions. Don't just tell her to breathe; breathe with her. Some women want you to count off the seconds; others don't. Be guided by her responses, even if they're a little impolite at the height of a contraction.

If she's having an epidural, your help will also be appreciated. See the 'What to expect during epidural placement' section, later in this chapter, for the do's and don'ts.

Transition labour

Transition, the hardest stage, is the last part of active labour. Transition lasts from 7 centimetres to full dilation, or 10 centimetres. If your partner has an epidural, this stage will probably breeze by, but if she's going natural, transition can be difficult. Transition can last anywhere from a few minutes in someone having a second or subsequent baby to a few hours in a woman having her first child. Typical side effects of transition include

- ✔ Shaking.
- ✔ Vomiting.
- ✔ Intermittent urges to push.

Second stage

Second-stage labour covers the first push to the final delivery and can last anywhere from two minutes to three-plus hours. Women with epidurals often push less effectively, and the midwife may let the baby 'labour down' without pushing if she's comfortable and the baby is doing okay.

Push, push, push!

Active pushing requires help from you, but don't actually push along with her, or you may have haemorrhoids the size of the baby after delivery. The midwife may ask you to help support your partner's legs or to support her back slightly.

The people in attendance at the delivery usually do lots of enthusiastic cheering when mum starts pushing. You'll find it easy to be enthusiastic when the baby's head finally begins to appear, although a little apprehension about how that big thing is going to make its way out of your partner's body is also normal.

Not all women are into the cheerleading scene, though, and actually prefer just to hear a single voice (yours) offering encouragement, or perhaps prefer no loud noises at all. If she looks aggravated during the cheers (beyond the effort of pushing), ask her what she wants. Then do it, and ask everyone else to comply.

Some delivery rooms have mirrors near the foot of the bed so that your partner can see what's going on. When your midwife or doctor takes their seat at the end of the delivery bed, she may block the mirror, but most mirrors can be adjusted so your partner has a better view if she wants it. Pushing is difficult with your eyes open, so she may not see much of the actual birth.

If you want to cut the cord, make your wishes known, although many practitioners will ask you automatically. If you're turning a little green, don't feel like you have to cut the cord. In fact, if you're turning a little green, please go and sit on the floor, or in a chair, so the staff don't have to tend to you.

Getting a little lightheaded during delivery is not a sign of weakness. Many guys don't eat enough while their partner is in labour, and you may be standing for several hours helping her push. Deliveries are very messy; vomit, poo and blood can make a pungent odour that can be hard to deal with, even for the most experienced labour and delivery staff. Try not to add to the mess by passing out and taking the delivery tray with you.

It's a miracle!

Birth is miraculous. There's no other way to put it. Even practitioners who have seen thousands of births are still awed by it at times. Watching a new human being come into the world is an amazing privilege, especially when he's *your* new human being.

Crying at deliveries isn't unusual. Of course the baby usually cries and family members often do too, but sometimes even the staff cry if they've become really attached to a particular couple. Don't expect your midwife or doctor to get all teary eyed, although it does happen in some cases.

Don't be surprised if your first feeling upon seeing your baby is dismay, either. New babies aren't always the most beautiful of creatures. (We discuss newborn peculiarities in Chapter 10.)

If the baby is okay, your practitioner may give him to your partner to hold and possibly to breastfeed, if she wants to try immediately. Some hospitals prefer to dry off, weigh and assess the baby before bringing him back to mum to nurse. Either way, within the first 15 minutes, the baby will be dried off, weighed and wrapped up so one or both of you can hold him or your partner can start nursing.

Wrapping things up after the birth

The placenta is usually delivered within 15 minutes of the birth. Contractions may accompany the loosening and passage of the placenta, but if your partner had an epidural, she may not notice. If the placenta doesn't pass within 15 minutes, some medical practitioners give additional medication to help loosen it or they gently tug on it. Both the medication and tugging can cause uncomfortable cramping. Other practitioners give the placenta more time to release on its own before starting more medical interventions.

Very rarely, a condition called placenta accrete occurs in which the placenta can't be removed from the uterine wall. In severe cases, a hysterectomy is done because the placenta can't be removed and severe bleeding often develops.

If your partner has a tear, or had an episiotomy to give the baby a little extra room and avoid a tear, the wound needs to be closed after the placenta is delivered. Stitching everything back together usually takes about 15 minutes. An injection of numbing medication is given before stitches are put in unless your partner is still completely numb from the epidural. If she didn't have an epidural, passing the placenta and stitching may be mildly uncomfortable or annoying.

Delivery and recovery now occur in the same room in many hospitals and birthing centres, so the bed will be refreshed and your partner's nightgown changed after the mechanics of the delivery are all taken care of. And she can eat! If she wants something special, you may be sent out to get what she wants, or, better yet, send one of her friends or her mum out so you can stay to admire your new family.

Helping baby right after delivery

If the baby doesn't breathe well at first (many don't, so don't panic), he may be taken right over to the warmer to be given a little oxygen. Don't worry; the staff will bring him back to your partner as soon as he's stable.

As normal as it is to ask a lot of questions and want to know exactly what's happening, try to stay on the sidelines so you're not interfering with your baby's care. You want the staff to focus on taking care of the baby, not talking to you.

Most issues that affect babies right after delivery are related to breathing. Not breathing inside the uterus to breathing on one's own is a big transition, and some babies take a few minutes to get the hang of it.

Oxygen may be given by *blow by*, which means a tube is placed near the baby's nose but not too close to his eyes. If he needs extra help, oxygen is given with a bag and mask connected to an oxygen source; the mask fits over his mouth and nose, and the staff squeeze the bag to force oxygen into the lungs.

If the baby doesn't pink up and start crying quickly, he may be taken to the special care unit for further evaluation. You will usually be welcome to accompany him and find out what's happening, but don't forget your partner, still lying on the bed feeling as confused and upset as you are and possibly getting sewn up at the same time. Make sure you keep her informed about what's happening and let her know you haven't forgotten about her. She may want you to follow the baby so you can report back and tell her what's going on.

Undergoing Common Labour Procedures

In the interests of making you familiar with all possible aspects of labour and delivery, some of the procedures you can expect to see during labour are detailed in the next sections.

Vaginal examinations

Vaginal examinations are often uncomfortable, especially when they're done during a contraction, but they're the only way to tell what's happening during labour. The cervix is checked for dilation, which is the only way to assess labour progression. Although your partner may not be overly fond of vaginal checks, you may love them because they give you new information to convey to friends and family in the waiting room or on the other end of the phone.

IVs

If you're delivering in a hospital, your partner may well have an *intravenous infusion*, or IV for short. The IV serves the following purposes:

- **Supplying fluids:** Many hospitals restrict fluids when labour begins, and getting dehydrated is easy when you're working extra hard and not taking anything in. If an epidural is given, prehydration is necessary to avoid a drop in blood pressure, which can decrease oxygen flow to the baby.

- **In case of caesarean delivery:** With the percentage of caesarean deliveries rising, a chance exists that your partner will end up having one. If the surgery is done as an emergency, with time being of the essence, having an IV already in place saves time.

- **Covering the hospital's legal obligations:** If a woman has serious bleeding, an emergency caesarean or just about any complication, an IV is necessary to give fluids to replace possible blood loss and maintain normal blood pressure, which often drops if spinal anaesthesia is given for the surgery.

After an IV is in place it shouldn't be terribly uncomfortable, so if it is, let your partner's midwife know. Sometimes just retaping the catheter so it's at a different angle helps with the discomfort. Women who want to walk without dragging around an IV pole or have a bath can have the IV hep-locked, which means the end is capped off and the bag of fluid detached. If needed, the hep-lock is flushed with solution to make sure it's still working before the bag is reattached.

Membrane ruptures

Although many women fear that their waters will break in an embarrassing location, like in the middle of the supermarket, only around 10 per cent of women's membranes rupture before labour starts. Often the membranes are broken by medical personnel using what looks like a crochet hook to snag the membranes and tear them. This procedure isn't painful for your partner or the baby.

Membranes are ruptured if your practitioner wants to check the fluid inside the sac for the presence of meconium (the baby's poo), a sign of potential stress, sometime before or during labour. Between 6 to 25 per cent of babies pass meconium before delivery; the older the meconium, the yellower and less particulate the fluid is. Newer meconium may be dark green, sticky and form particles that can be sucked into the baby's lungs, causing respiratory problems at birth. The presence of either old or new meconium can cause respiratory problems at birth, so the fluid is always checked for meconium as soon as the membranes rupture.

If meconium is present, your practitioner will suck out the baby's nose and mouth as soon as the head is delivered to decrease the chance of inhalation. Keep in mind, however, that meconium can be inhaled before birth; there's no way to prevent this from happening because babies take practice breaths while still in the uterus. Most of the time, the baby clears the meconium from the lungs, and no problems ensue, but it can cause severe lung infection and problems with circulation that require mechanical ventilation until the lungs heal, usually within a few days.

The membrane may also be ruptured to try to speed up labour (although labour doesn't always go faster as a result), or so that internal monitoring devices can be placed. (See the next section for more about the different ways in which your baby's heartbeat can be monitored before birth.)

Rupturing membranes can lead to harder, more painful contractions that don't actually speed up the process, so ask your medical practitioner why it is necessary if you have concerns about it.

Foetal monitoring

Foetal monitoring devices record the foetal heart rate and the frequency and duration of the contractions. Don't let yourself become so enamoured with the technology that you forget about the person at the other end! Many men love gadgets and start watching the monitor like it was the sports channel. (See the nearby sidebar 'Understanding foetal heart rates' for more on what's normal and what's not.)

Monitoring your partner and the baby externally

External monitoring systems consist of two recording devices fastened around your partner's stomach and plugged into a foetal monitor, which provides a continuous printout of the foetal heart rate and the contractions. The monitor records the duration of contractions and the time between them but doesn't tell you the strength of the contraction. Each contraction resembles a hill or a bell-shaped curve, starting low, rising slowly and then returning to baseline. Because the device sits on your partner's abdomen, attached with a belt, her body shape and position can affect how the contractions look on the monitor. Contractions that look like very large mountains on the monitor don't always indicate really strong contractions, and tiny hills don't mean the contractions aren't very strong.

The external foetal heart monitor tracks and records the foetal heart rate but has some limitations as well. It doesn't record the baby's exact heartbeat, but an average of beats. Variability, the difference in heart rate over a certain time period, can't be determined by external monitors, and beat-to-beat variability can help ascertain how well the baby is handling labour.

A heartbeat that stays the same with little variation may indicate that the baby is stressed. Short periods of decreased variability also occur when the baby is asleep. (And yes, babies do take short naps during labour!) The foetal heart rate may also have a short period of minimal beat-to-beat variability if your partner gets a dose of narcotic pain medication.

The external monitor also can't always distinguish between mum's heart rate and baby's. If your partner has a rapid heartbeat because of fever, anxiety or other reasons, or if the baby has bradycardia, an extremely low heart rate, it may not be obvious that the external monitor isn't recording the right heartbeat.

Monitoring internally

Internal monitors resolve the shortcomings of external monitors by giving more accurate information. Internal contraction monitors are inserted directly into the uterus, which makes them able to record the exact strength of each contraction. You may be disappointed to watch those huge mountains that appeared to be very strong contractions shrink down to little blips on the monitor, indicating that the uterus is contracting only mildly, or you may be excited to see the opposite.

Internal foetal monitors fasten a tiny wire into the baby's scalp that records the exact foetal heart rate. This ensures that variability displayed is an accurate representation of the foetal heartbeat. An internal monitor can also differentiate maternal and foetal heart rates, if it's difficult to tell whose heart rate is recording on the external monitor.

Some centres use internal monitors routinely, while others use them only if they're having trouble picking up the heart rate or assessing the contractions. Internal monitor complications occur rarely, and include infection at the site of insertion or haematoma, a large bruise.

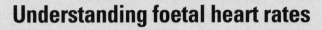

Understanding foetal heart rates

A normal foetal heart rate ranges from 110 to 160 beats per minute (BPM). Variations in the heart rate often occur for a short period of time before returning to baseline. Babies all have different baselines, so a heart rate of 115 BPM may be normal for one baby, but *bradycardic*, or unusually slow, for one whose baseline is 160 BPM.

Brief increases in the heart rate are called accelerations. They occur when the baby moves, if he runs a temperature or if he develops an infection. If the baby's heart beats too fast, your medical provider may say the baby is *tachycardic*, or *tachy*. Tachycardia can become dangerous because less oxygen is pumped out of the heart with each beat.

Brief drops in the heart rate often occur at the peak of the contraction and are caused by temporary pressure on the baby's head during active labour as the baby descends into the birth canal. Bradycardia may also be caused by cord compression, if the baby compresses the cord with some part of his body and oxygen flow is temporarily decreased.

Bradycardia that lasts just a few seconds is not considered alarming, but bradycardia that lasts after the end of a contraction or that starts after the peak of the contraction, recovering shortly after the end of the contraction, can indicate decreased blood flow through the placenta.

Any unusual change in the foetal heart rate can be better assessed with continuous monitoring with an internal foetal monitor, which records an exact representation of the baby's heartbeat.

Coping with Labour Pain

Although you and your partner discussed pain medication options before the big day (and we discuss making the decision on pain medication in Chapter 8), nothing is written in stone when labour actually starts. A staunch au naturel supporter may find herself asking for an epidural the minute she hits the labour ward, and a woman who was sure she's epidural material may find herself breathing through labour and deciding she'd rather do without one. Don't ever be surprised by the decisions of a labouring woman.

Enduring it: Going natural

Going natural was all the rage in the 1970s but fell out of favour when epidural anaesthesia became available in all but the smallest hospitals. Natural delivery still does have some advantages, and good reasons exist to consider an unmedicated delivery. Your partner may decide to go natural for the following reasons:

- Babies whose mums haven't received medication may be more alert and may nurse better. Medication does cross the placenta to the foetus before delivery.

- Moving around during labour is easier if you're not medicated. Epidural anaesthesia usually keeps you in bed, although 'walking epidurals' are offered by some hospitals.

- Pushing is easier without an epidural, although some hospitals let an epidural wear down enough for mum to be able to push.

- Water therapy can't be utilised if you have epidural anaesthesia.

- Going through labour unmedicated can be an empowering experience.

- Some women have bad reactions to medications in general and don't want to take anything they don't really need.

One good thing about going natural is that with a first labour, it's usually never too late to change your mind and request an epidural.

Dulling it: Sedation (no, not for you)

Sedation takes the edge off labour without numbing the lower part of the body. IV administration takes effect quickly and lasts one to two hours.

Sedation may be given if it's too early in the labour to give epidural anaesthesia. Sedation can take the edge off the pain and help your partner get a little sleep, but it can also slow contractions in some cases.

Because sedation can reach the baby, narcotics and narcotic-type medications often are not given if delivery is expected within the hour because the baby may not breathe well.

Blotting it out: Epidurals

Epidural anaesthesia consists of medications given through a catheter placed in the spinal canal. The benefit of epidurals is obvious: they decrease pain. But they also have other benefits as well, in some cases. For example,

> ✔ Epidurals can help a tense mum relax. Tension can slow labour; women who are especially tense may benefit from an epidural to help them loosen up a bit.
>
> ✔ Epidurals provide continuous pain relief. In many cases, a continuous infusion of medication prevents the medication from wearing off.

Medications used in epidurals

Several different types of medication are used in epidural anaesthesia. Anaesthetics such as lidocaine or bupivacaine may be combined with narcotics such as fentanyl or morphine. Narcotics decrease the amount of local anaesthetics needed to achieve adequate comfort. Narcotics given in an epidural don't cause drowsiness the way sedatives do.

What to expect during epidural placement

An epidural can be given at any stage of labour, but usually isn't given in very early labour because it can slow progress. Some doctors will start a drug to induce labour when epidural anaesthesia is given in early labour.

A large amount of IV fluid, approximately one bag, is infused rapidly to offset the drop in blood pressure that may occur with epidural anaesthesia. This infusion can be uncomfortable because the fluid is at room temperature and feels cold.

Dads are very much in demand during epidural placement to give mum a person to lean on so she can get into the proper 'curled shrimp' position for catheter placement (see Figure 9-1). The epidural catheter is placed into the epidural place on the midback by inserting a metal needle into the epidural space and then threading the catheter through the needle. Only the soft plastic catheter remains in the back. She must remain sitting up and still, even through contractions, for a period of five to ten minutes while the catheter is placed.

After the catheter is taped in place, the anaesthetist assists her back to a lying-down position and assesses her blood pressure and comfort level for several minutes. In many hospitals, the epidural catheter is attached to an infusion pump that delivers a continuous infusion during labour to help maintain adequate pain relief.

If you feel at all shaky or nervous while your partner receives the epidural, or if you start to get lightheaded from standing in one position too long, ask someone else to take over supporting mum so you can sit down before you fall down.

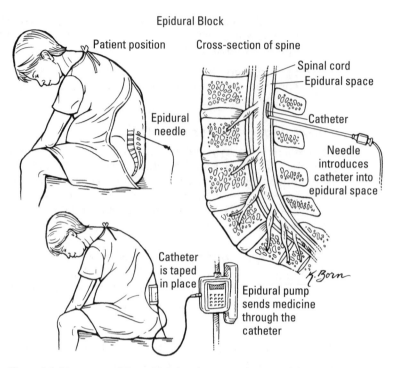

Figure 9-1: Placement of the epidural catheter requires remaining curled up and still for a short period.

Sometimes placing the catheter is difficult as a result of your partner's anatomy, and more than one attempt may be necessary. This situation isn't anyone's fault, and getting the catheter correctly placed is important, so you can help by staying calm and keeping your partner calm, too.

When the catheter is in place, a test dose is given and your partner's blood pressure is carefully assessed, because epidural anaesthesia can cause blood pressure to drop. She has to wear an automatic blood-pressure cuff on her arm for a short period, and she may find this very uncomfortable. If her blood pressure is low, she may be tilted slightly to her left side.

Possible side effects of an epidural

Following are some of the side effects of epidural anaesthesia:

   ✔ **A rise in temperature:** It's difficult to tell whether infection or the epidural is causing a rise in temperature, so intravenous antibiotics can sometimes be given to avoid complications in

case an infection is present. Any time mum runs a temperature, the foetus may also develop one, from the increase in
uterine temperature.

✔ **Nausea and/or vomiting:** These symptoms may also occur in
labours without epidurals.

✔ **Shivering:** The fluid infusion or the epidural can cause shivering. Your partner will appreciate extra blankets, especially if
they're warmed.

✔ **Hot spots:** Sometimes women have an area that doesn't 'take'
to the epidural, and they need to change positions so that the
anaesthesia goes to a different area and numbs the nerves
that haven't been numbed well. In the worst-case scenario,
the epidural may need to be placed again.

✔ **Difficulty urinating:** Most women can't urinate properly after
the epidural is given, and a full bladder can get in the way
of the baby's head and slow the pushing stage of labour. A
catheter may be placed to drain urine, or the bladder may be
emptied intermittently.

Deviating From Your Birth Plan/Vision

Everyone has some vision of how labour is going to go, even if it
isn't committed to paper. But most labours don't follow the book,
or the birth plan. Knowing this ahead of time helps you avoid serious disappointment. Consider the birth plan as a guideline of what
you would like to happen, with the proviso that mum's and baby's
well-being come first.

Some women feel guilty about taking pain medication in labour if
they were gung-ho to go natural before delivery. If your partner
wants to take pain medication but is hesitating because she feels
like she's letting the birth plan – or you – down, encourage her to
follow her instincts. Remind her that no one knows what labour is
like until she's in it, and that most women do end up taking pain
medication in labour. After all, labour hurts!

On the other hand, your partner may have gone from au naturel
woman to 'give me the drugs!' seemingly in the blink of an eye,
and you may be the one having a hard time with it and trying to
encourage her to stick to the plan. Don't do it. Encouragement is
fine if she's just going through a rough spot in transition, for example, but if she's made her decision, your job is to support her in it.

You may have devised the birth plan together, but she's the one going through labour, not you.

If your partner ends up having a caesarean or if the baby has any type of problem, large or small, she may feel that something she did in labour caused the problem. Assure her that this is not the case (because it won't be). Things go wrong in labour that are no one's fault; they can't be predicted or, in most cases, prevented. Your job is to tell her that she did exactly what she should have and that she has no reason for regrets. And if you have any niggling doubts about the wisdom of her labour choices, keep them to yourself.

Having a Caesarean

Caesarean sections now comprise around a quarter of all deliveries in the UK (compared to just over a tenth in the 1980s). Although having a caesarean involves major surgery, the operation is generally safe for your partner and the baby. However, babies born by caesarean section may retain more fluid in the respiratory tract than babies born vaginally, and the fluid can be aspirated into the lungs, causing breathing difficulties.

Maternal complications such as infection, complications from the anaesthetic, blood clots and excessive bleeding can also occur, as with any surgery.

Scheduled caesareans

Caesareans may be scheduled ahead of time if you know your partner's going to need one. Knowing she's going to have a caesarean ahead of time helps you to get things ready for her homecoming, knowing that she's going to be extremely sore as well as tired. Your partner may not want to navigate stairs for the first week afterward, and won't be able to drive for several weeks.

Reasons for planned caesareans

Reasons for a scheduled caesarean include previous caesarean delivery and abnormal foetal position, such as breech (feet first) or transverse (sideways) lie. Most of the time, but not always, these are determined ahead of time, but babies have been known to switch position just a few days before delivery.

Occasionally, women ask for a medically unnecessary caesarean delivery. Some doctors will perform these procedures, but having surgery you don't need is never a good idea. Caesarean delivery is riskier for the baby because fluid doesn't get squeezed out of the lungs before delivery, setting up potential respiratory difficulties.

Multiples are almost always delivered by caesarean, even though twins who are both vertex (head down) can certainly be delivered vaginally. However, after the first twin is delivered, there's an abundance of room in the uterus, and the second twin may turn sideways with the joy of having all that space to himself, necessitating a caesarean for baby B. No mother wants to experience both a vaginal delivery and a caesarean with all the attendant discomforts on the same day, so most twins are scheduled for a caesarean section.

Setting the date

Choosing your baby's birth date can be exciting, but consider the following caveats:

✔ Don't choose a Saturday or Sunday if possible. There may be fewer staff on duty at the weekend.

✔ Don't expect to bypass the last three weeks of pregnancy with an early delivery date. More practitioners are trying to schedule caesareans no earlier than 38 weeks, to avoid preterm (before 37 weeks) delivery and potential complications.

✔ Understand that the baby may come before your scheduled date. The baby hasn't read your birth plan and doesn't know that you want him to be born on an auspicious date, and he may decide to show up a week earlier.

✔ Realise that having an 8 a.m. surgery time scheduled doesn't always mean your surgery will be at 8 a.m. Emergency cases can bump you off the schedule, which is understandable, so don't get too upset if you're delayed because someone else's operation needs to be done first.

Unplanned caesarean delivery

A large percentage of caesareans are unplanned, with the most common reason cited for them as 'failure to progress', which means labour wasn't progressing as expected. This can mean a baby too large for the pelvis, an unusual maternal anatomy or a doctor who is getting concerned about how things are going.

If labour goes on too long, complications such as infection become more likely, and doing a caesarean is often less stressful than waiting for the situation to possibly deteriorate.

Foetal distress is an undeniable reason for an unplanned caesarean, although true foetal distress is different from potential foetal distress that could possibly worsen if labour goes on. True foetal distress is marked by a run down the corridor at top speed, minimal surgery preparation and often general anaesthesia because it's the quickest way to put mum to sleep.

Potential foetal distress or mild distress usually results in a more leisurely trip to the operating theatre and a much calmer atmosphere, because the baby isn't in any real danger yet. And because you don't want him to reach that point, a caesarean can be the best option. Trust your obstetrician; if he says your partner needs a caesarean, go with it.

What to expect before the operation

Certain procedures must be done before a caesarean delivery. Normally, a catheter is placed in the bladder to keep it empty so it won't be injured during the surgery. If your partner already has an epidural, she won't even feel the catheter placement; if she doesn't, she may be mildly uncomfortable during the procedure.

A preparatory mini-shave is done (if she hasn't already done it herself) to eliminate hair where the incision goes. Most caesarean scars are known as a bikini cut, a horizontal lower abdominal incision (see Figure 9-2). Occasionally a vertical skin incision is done if the baby or babies lie in a position that makes him – or them – difficult to reach, or if the surgery has to be done very rapidly.

Your partner may be given medications to reduce the chance of nausea and to neutralise stomach acids in case of vomiting and possible aspiration into the lungs. She'll also be given an intravenous line if she doesn't already have one. If spinal anaesthesia is used for the procedure, fluid will be quickly infused, which can feel very cold. Also, an adequate amount of fluid is necessary to keep blood pressure from dropping after the caesarean.

Your partner may be taken into the operating room by herself while you get dressed in a sterile outfit. When you're allowed in, you'll probably be given a seat right near her head so you can talk to her and support her without getting in anyone's way. Keeping the operative area sterile is extremely important during surgery, and the staff will take care to make sure you don't inadvertently contaminate anything.

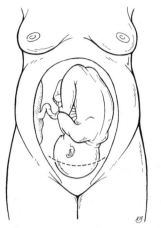 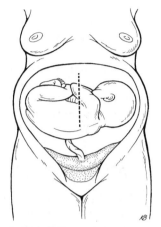

a. Low transverse   b. Classical

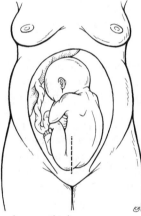

c. Low vertical

Figure 9-2: Most caesarean incisions are done just above the pubic hairline.

What to expect during the surgery

When the surgery actually gets underway, removing the baby takes between five and ten minutes. You won't be able to see much, because a sterile sheet is placed between your partner's head and the rest of her body. When the baby is delivered, he may be brought close to your partner so she can see him, but she won't be able to nurse immediately or do any type of skin-to-skin contact because of the sterile operating field.

If general anaesthesia isn't used, your partner may feel tugging during the surgery. This is normal, but she may need lots of reassurance that it's okay.

Because babies born by caesarean have an increased risk of complications, a paediatrician may be present for the delivery. You'll be allowed to walk over to the warmer to see the baby, and in many hospitals, after the baby is weighed and cleaned, he'll be given to you to hold next to your partner.

Getting past disappointment

When you have the baby, you have him; it doesn't really matter how he got here. Your partner may not see it that way, though, and she may mourn the loss of the 'perfect' labour and delivery and feel like she failed the labour test. With so many women having caesareans today, this feeling of failure is less common than it used to be, but if you and your partner had your hearts set on a certain labour scenario, a deviation from the script can be upsetting.

You can be a big help by accentuating the positives in the situation, by reminding her how well she handled the change in plans and how she put the baby's needs before her wishes.

Understanding why certain procedures were necessary can be very important in helping new mothers 'grieve' the loss of a perfect delivery. Ask if you can speak to the person who delivered your baby so that you and your partner can ask lingering questions about why the delivery went the way it did.

Chapter 10

Caring for Your Newborn

· ·

· ·

*W*alking out of the hospital door with a newborn baby who is still basically a stranger to you can be a scary experience. Getting to know your baby is a process that takes time. Fortunately you'll be putting in lots of time with this demanding stranger, and before you know it, you'll feel as if you've known this marvellous little person all your life. In this chapter we talk you through the seemingly mundane tasks that help you build a lifetime relationship with your new baby.

Knowing What to Expect When Baby is Born

Newborns don't look anything like the smooth-skinned, dimpled, smiling babies on TV. A new baby emerges from nine months in a dark, watery environment, and her skin shows it. She squints like she's just emerged from a cave. Although your newborn may not look exactly like the baby in your idealised dreams, she'll look perfect to you – at least after you get used to her in a day or two.

Looking at newborns

What should you expect when your newborn is put into your arms for the first time? Well, newborn babies have the following characteristics:

✔ **Small:** The average baby weighs around 7 pounds (3kg) and is 20 inches (50cm) long. The reality of how small and fragile a newborn seems won't hit you until the first time you hold her.

✔ **Red and covered with – what's that white stuff?** Newborns are amazingly red. They come out a dark red and then turn a lighter red, which gradually fades to a normal skin colour over a few days. Many newborns are coated, especially in the creases, with *vernix*, a creamy substance that protected newborn skin in water.

✔ **Wrinkled and peeling:** Since she just spent nine months immersed in water, her entire skin has the equivalent of washing-up hands, and as soon as she begins to dry out, her skin wrinkles because it's no longer waterlogged. Her skin will crack and peel, especially around the bendable joints like the ankles and wrists.

✔ **Cone-headed:** You thought the cone heads weren't real, until you met your new baby. If your partner pushed for any amount of time, or if the baby was delivered by vacuum extraction, the baby's head may be pointed at the back, or she may have a little cone cup, like a jaunty little hat, to the side of her head. The baby's head will become round in a week or so. Caesarean babies usually escape the cone-head look.

✔ **Spotted, dotted and blotched:** Newborns often have a variety of blotches, splotches, whiteheads and other marks that will fade over time. *Milia* look like little whiteheads on the baby's nose, chin and forehead. Don't squeeze them; they'll disappear on their own. The majority of babies of Asian, East Indian and African descent have what look like black and blue marks on their legs or buttocks, called *Mongolian spots*, which fade with time. Red blotches on the back of the neck, eyelids and between the eyes, called *stork bites*, are immature blood vessels that also disappear with time.

✔ **Not very well put together:** Newborns often seem like they may fall apart if a strong wind comes along. Their heads wobble alarmingly, and their arms and legs shoot off in all directions when they're startled. No wonder midwives wrap them up tight in blankets.

✔ **A bit, uh, out of proportion:** You may be saying, 'That's my boy!' but baby boys may have overlarge genitals as a result of fluid retention, trauma during delivery and hormonal influences. This condition is temporary. Girls often have swollen genitalia as well, but it's less noticeable. Also, girls may pass a few drops of blood from the vagina.

✔ **Swollen breasts:** Because of maternal hormones, both baby boys and girls often have swollen breasts that may actually produce a few drops of milk. This condition disappears within a few days.

✔ **May demonstrate no family resemblance:** Before you ask your partner whether the baby is yours, rest assured that many newborns have puffiness and swelling around the eyes, and the yellow tinge of jaundice that many babies have after the first day or two may have you convinced that someone has a lot of explaining to do. Puffiness will improve daily, and by the end of the week, you won't be able to stop telling everyone how much the baby looks like you.

Rating the reflexes

Newborns are active from the minute they're born. Your baby will yawn, grimace and even seem to smile a little. (Yes, the smiles are really caused by wind at this stage, just like your mother says.) Babies also have certain reflex actions that are normal at birth. Your medical practitioner will assess the baby to make sure these reflexes are present. Lack of normal reflexes can indicate a problem that should be investigated. They include the following tests:

✔ **Babinski reflex:** When the bottom of her foot is stroked, the big toe rises and the other toes fan out. The Babinski reflex lasts for around two years.

✔ **Grasp reflex:** If the baby's palm is stroked, she closes her fingers, a reflex that lasts several months.

✔ **The Moro, or startle, reflex:** Your baby tremors slightly, throws back her head and flails her arms and legs away from her side in response to a sudden movement or loud noise. The Moro reflex lasts five or six months before disappearing.

✔ **Rooting reflex:** Stroking the corner of the baby's mouth makes her turn toward the touch; this helps her find the breast or bottle for feeding.

✔ **Step reflex:** When her foot touches a solid surface, she appears to step, lifting one foot and then the other.

✔ **Sucking reflex:** When an object touches the roof of the baby's mouth, she begins to suck. This reflex doesn't develop until around 32 weeks of pregnancy and isn't fully developed until 36 weeks.

✔ **Tonic neck reflex (TNR):** If the baby's head turns to the side, her arm on that side stretches out and the opposite arm bends at the elbow, which makes her look like she's fencing. The TNR lasts six to seven months.

Feeding a Newborn

Every baby needs to be fed, but the sheer number of choices to be made about feeding may have you begging your partner to consider nothing but breastfeeding for at least the next year. However, though breastfeeding is best for the baby, it may not be best for your partner.

While your opinion is probably valued, the final decision about breastfeeding is absolutely, unquestionably, your partner's. Many women just aren't comfortable with breastfeeding, and a woman who isn't comfortable usually won't do it well. Sure, breast is best, but bottle-feeding is a perfectly adequate method of feeding.

A number of considerations go into the decision to breast- or bottle-feed. If your partner has even the slightest interest, breastfeeding for the first few days so the baby receives *colostrum*, the first fluids produced, is a good way to start. Colostrum contains many nutrients and antibodies that are good for the baby. If your partner hates it, she can stop at any time, but she may love it! If she stops breastfeeding, though, it's hard, but not at all impossible, to get the milk flowing again. See Chapter 11 for more on making the decision to breastfeed.

Choosing to breastfeed

If your partner decides to breastfeed, you may be breathing a sigh of relief that the night-time duties won't fall to you – but not so fast! Breastfed babies usually eat more frequently than bottle-fed babies because breast milk is more easily digested. If the baby is sleeping in your bed, or even across the room, you'll probably be awake at 12 a.m., 3 a.m. and 6 a.m., too.

Even if you normally sleep like the dead and wouldn't wake up if the *Titanic* floated through your bedroom, getting up and offering support for at least one of the night feeds can be a wonderful contribution to your partner and make you feel closer to your baby. Get your partner a drink, help her get into a comfortable position and talk to her if she wants conversation. Late-night talks are conducive to confidences and discussions you may not have time for during the day.

If you're working full-time, getting up in the night is hard but worth it. Getting to know your new little person and your partner better is worth the sacrifice, and this time too shall pass, faster than you can imagine.

Getting started

Although breastfeeding seems like it should be easy and natural, it isn't always. Many women today have no role models for breast-feeding; their mums may not have breastfed, their friends may not be doing it and you're not much help, either. Most hospitals have specialist nurses to help new mums get started on breastfeeding. Some also offer at-home visits if needed.

Also, the National Childbirth Trust (NCT) provides breastfeeding counsellors who can be contacted at any time and will come to your home.

And of course, books like *Breastfeeding For Dummies*, by Sharon Perkins and Carol Vannais (Wiley) cover everything you need to know and are available for consultation day and night! The most common problems encountered with breastfeeding include:

- **Latch-on problems:** Women with large or flat nipples often have a difficult time getting the baby to latch on. This is frus-trating for mum and baby alike, and often ends with both in tears. If the baby isn't properly latched, she won't get a good milk supply. Patience, and in some cases, using a nipple shield, which fits over the nipple to give the baby something to grasp onto if nipples are very flat, can conquer latch-on problems.

- **Supply issues:** Most women have ample milk supply starting around the third day after delivery, but some need supple-ments to increase it. Drinking plenty of fluids, getting enough rest and eating herbs like fenugreek can help increase supply. Before a good milk supply is established, supplementing the baby's diet with formula or pumping rather than nursing is discouraged, because sucking increases the supply. Pumping isn't as effective as a baby's suck at stimulating milk supply. Breast milk is the original supply-and-demand system.

- **Parental anxiety:** Many new parents are obsessed with their baby's weight. Breastfeeding can frustrate parents who want to know how much milk the baby is getting at each feed. However, you can still measure her intake if you have baby scales; just weigh the baby before and after a feed and com-pare. Don't change her clothes, not even her nappy, or the weight won't be accurate. Baby scales can save the sanity of weight-obsessed parents.

Supplemental bottles

After the milk supply is well established, supplemental bottles of formula or pumped breast milk can be given. Bottle-feeding is a nice way for you to be able to feed and bond with the baby occasionally, and it gives your partner a chance to get out of the house or actually take an uninterrupted shower. Decreasing the number of nursing times a day reduces the milk supply, though, so don't overdo the supplemental bottles.

Don't be surprised if the baby doesn't quite understand what to do with the bottle at first. Bottle-feeding and breastfeeding require completely different tongue positioning and techniques on the baby's part. Some babies refuse supplemental bottles, which can be a problem if your partner becomes unwell or for some reason can't breastfeed. While you can feed a recalcitrant breastfeeder with an eyedropper, it certainly isn't fun for either of you. Some medical practitioners recommend an occasional supplemental bottle after nursing is well established so the baby gets used to taking an occasional bottle.

Many dads are a little envious of the closeness of the breastfeeding relationship and enjoy skin-to-skin contact while they feed the baby. Others find this just too weird. Whichever camp you're in, supplemental bottles can give you time to study your baby's face in detail and revel in the miracle you've created.

Pumping

Pumping to fill a supplemental bottle or if your partner goes back to work is easier than it used to be. Your partner can use an electric pump that's more efficient than the old bicycle horn-type pumps. A really good pump can be very pricy but is worth it if your partner is going to use it a lot. Pumping is nowhere near as efficient as nursing, so the amount produced may be much less than you think it should be. This difference is normal and not a sign that the baby isn't getting enough milk.

Pumped milk should be stored in feed-sized amounts, especially if you're freezing it, because you don't want to thaw out more than you'll use at one time. Use plastic or glass containers with well-fitted tops, but avoid anything containing bisphenol A (BPA). Collection bags made specifically for freezing breast milk are ideal.

Don't use plastic bags or bags from disposable bottles, which may leak or contain substances that affect the nutrients in breast milk.

Breast milk can be stored at room temperature for up to six hours, in the refrigerator for up to eight days and in the freezer for up to 12 months.

Bottle-feeding basics

Bottle-feeding has never been more complicated. Not only do you have to choose a formula and a nipple type, you have to worry about the materials the bottle is made of. Recent reports about the high levels of bisphenol-A (BPA),a chemical used in plastics, released when bottles are heated in the microwave or dishwasher has made choosing a bottle type more difficult. At least bottles no longer need to be sterilised by boiling them in a saucepan: ask your mum or grandma about how much fun that used to be!

Winning the bottle battle

Once upon a time, all baby bottles were made of glass. Then parents got tired of being hit over the head with glass bottles, and everyone worried about glass bottles breaking when the baby threw them out of the cot, so plastic bottles were invented about two minutes after the invention of plastic. Not only were they lighter and unbreakable, but they also came in pretty colours.

Then bottle manufacturers decided to mix things up a bit. Now bottles and nipples are no longer interchangeable, and bottle 'systems' sometimes include plastic liners and inserts that reduce air intake and, hopefully, colic. Every bottle has to be used with its own system, and parents have to decide which works best for their baby.

Studies have shown cause for concern about plastic bottles releasing the harmful chemical BPA when heated. Some parents have switched back to glass, but manufacturers now create BPA-free plastic bottle systems. If you have older bottles and they're not BPA free, get rid of them. Spending more money on another whole bottle system is painful, but it's better than worrying about poisoning your child every time you warm a bottle in the microwave.

Choosing a formula

After you pick your bottles, you can start worrying about which formula to use. The array is truly formidable. For starters, you have to consider powder versus concentrate versus readymade. Following are the advantages and disadvantages of each type:

- ✔ **Ready to serve** can be very convenient for travel, if you use one carton at a feeding. However, this method is out of the question for everyday use for most people, because a month's supply is equal to the national budget of a small European country.

- ✔ **Concentrate** comes in small tins, and you dilute it with water before feeding. It's easy to use but more expensive than powder, though it's cheaper than ready to serve.

✔ **Powder** is the cheapest of the three options. If you're out of the house, it's easy to put the powder in a bottle and just fill with warm water when the baby's ready to eat. On the downside, it clumps and takes more effort to shake smooth, a consideration at 4 a.m. when any effort seems like too much. Shaking the bottle to mix increases the bubbles and air inside the bottle, which can cause wind, so if your baby is already prone to wind, powder formula may not be for you.

After you decide on the form of your formula, it's time to choose one. Doing so won't be easy; about a hundred different formulas are on the market, all claiming to be the best (although most grudgingly acknowledge that breastfeeding is also very good). Following are the general categories of formulas:

✔ **Regular:** Regular formula is made from cow's milk and contains 20 calories per ounce. Regular formula is usually fortified with iron. Some are also fortified with long-chain polyunsaturated fats that they claim enhance eye and brain development, but these claims are not well substantiated.

✔ **Enhanced:** Enhanced formula, often used for premature or failure-to-thrive babies, contains 24 calories per ounce.

✔ **Soya:** Soya-based formulas may be used by parents wanting to avoid animal proteins. However, soya contains oestrogen, and some studies show that too much soya can be harmful to infants and children. Make sure to do your research before you switch to soya.

✔ **Hypoallergenic:** Babies who are allergic to lactose or soya may need protein hydrolysate formulas, which are easier to digest.

Preparing a bottle

The hardest part of preparing some bottles is putting the 'system' together. Some bottles have inserts to put in, and others have little bags to put in place that hold the formula.

To make a bottle, read the instructions on the formula label. For powder, you mix a certain number of scoops with a certain amount of water, sometimes a foggy concept in the middle of the night. Concentrates are usually diluted 1:1, and ready-to-serve formulas don't get diluted at all.

Never try to 'stretch' formula by adding more water than usual or by adding water to ready-to-serve formulas. You may deprive your baby of essential nutrition by doing so.

If you want to use well water, have a sample of it tested to make sure it doesn't contain high levels of nitrates or other minerals. Boiling well water concentrates nitrates instead of removing them, so it isn't recommended.

Knowing how much formula is enough

When your baby is brand new, she probably won't take more than 2 or 3 ounces at a time. The most important thing about bottle-feeding is not to force the last drop down your child's throat. With childhood obesity at an all-time high and a major health concern, the last thing you want to do is overfeed your child from an early age.

On the other hand, if she drains the bottle and acts like she's still hungry, give her a little more. Babies aren't machines, and they don't take the same amount of formula at each feed. When she stops sucking and tries to push the bottle out of her mouth, she's had enough.

Changing Nappies

Changing nappies is the task new parents are probably least excited about. If you and your partner find yourselves playing 'rock, paper, scissors' to determine which of you gets stuck changing the runny yellow poo that's overflowed out of the nappy and on to the babygro, your shirt and the new leather sofa, you're normal.

Nappy duty isn't fun, but it is necessary an appalling number of times a day when your baby is new, so rest assured you'll both get plenty of experience.

Cleaning baby boys

Boys and girls really are different when it comes to nappy changing. When dealing with a baby boy, the worst part is projectile urination. You can easily avoid it if you remember to keep the penis covered at all times. A few good shots to the eye will quickly reinforce your memory.

In uncircumcised boys the foreskin doesn't retract, or pull back easily, before the age of one year or even longer. Up to this point, only the outside of the foreskin should be cleaned. When it can be retracted, gently push it back as far as it will go, which isn't very far, and clean with only water. Return the foreskin to its normal position afterward. If the foreskin becomes red or swollen, have your GP take a look to make sure he doesn't have an infection.

Cleaning baby girls

Baby girls aren't likely to spray the room when you remove their nappy, but they have their own set of problems. Keep these points in mind when changing a baby girl:

- Girls have lots of creases, and getting all of them clean is difficult. A runny, pooey nappy goes everywhere. Use moistened wipes or cotton balls to make sure you remove all the stool.

- Girls are more likely to have urinary tract infections because of the proximity of the anus and vagina to the urethra, so it's really important to make sure the whole area is clean.

- Always wipe from front to back. Doing so helps to avoid introducing faecal matter into the vaginal area, which can cause infections.

- Don't be too gentle. Make sure to thoroughly wipe the opening of the vagina or it can close up. If that happens you will have to apply a steroid cream to help reopen it, or, even worse, have it surgically reopened.

Bathing Basics

Few things strike fear into the hearts of inexperienced parents like the first bath. Take a squirmy baby, soap her all over to make her incredibly difficult to hold on to and then put her in a tub of water. Sounds like a recipe for disaster, or at the very least, parental heart failure, but it doesn't have to be. Many hospitals now do a trial run bath to make sure you won't drown the poor child at the first go, but even the least experienced new dad can learn to give the bath. Remember these suggestions when getting ready for baby's first bath:

1. **Get your supplies ready first.**

   Nothing makes a bath more difficult than getting the bath run, the baby undressed and the towel laid out and realising you forgot to get the soap, or the lotion, or the nappy. No, the baby doesn't wear the nappy in the bath; you need it ready the minute you take the baby out, though, especially if your baby's a boy, unless you want an eyeful of wee.

2. **Put the baby in a comfortable spot.**

   Undressing her on the toilet lid may seem like a good idea if you're bathing her in the basin, or on the counter if you're bathing her in a little baby bath, but those surfaces are cold and hard, even with a towel over them, and they

may be riddled with germs. Get her ready on the changing
table or bed; take off everything except the nappy (wee,
remember?) and bring her into the bathroom wrapped in
the towel.

3. **Hold the baby and fill the bath, or have your partner
   handle one of those jobs.**

   Bath water for the baby should be 90 to100 °F (32.2 to
   37.8 °C). You can monitor the temperature to make sure it
   isn't too hot or isn't getting too cold with cute little floating
   bath toys that have built-in thermometers. If you're using
   a basin, pad it by lining it with a towel. A towel also helps
   reduce the slipperiness of a baby bath.

4. **Before putting the baby into the bath, wet a flannel and
   squirt the baby soap onto it.**

   This way you don't have to do it while you try to hold the
   baby in the water at the same time.

5. **Undo the nappy tabs, then whip off the nappy and put
   the baby in the water.**

   Don't give the baby time to do anything dastardly.

6. **Don't expect the baby to enjoy this new experience at
   first.**

   Yes, she spent nine months in water, but she's forgotten
   already, and your inexperienced hands aren't supporting
   her as well as the uterus did. Some baby baths have a little
   sling or are curved to support the baby. Otherwise, support her head and neck with your hand, or the crook of
   your arm, if you're well co-ordinated.

7. **Wash the baby with the soapy flannel, starting at her
   head and working your way down.**

   Yes, just like you'd wash the wall, or the car. The genitalia should be the last part you wash. When you get to
   the bottom (literally), use a clean flannel if it seems more
   hygienic to you.

8. **Rinse her off with a clean flannel.**

9. **Lift her out of the water and wrap the towel around her.**

   A towel with a little hood helps keep her warm and makes
   her look like an adorable elf. Don't admire her too long,
   because you need to get her nappy back on – quickly.

10. **Carry her to the changing surface, where the fresh nappy
    is already laid out. To keep her warm, keep the towel
    over the top half of her body while you put the nappy on.**

11. **Dry her off gently and dress her.**

    Babies have delicate skin, so don't rub too hard with the towel.

12. **Now collapse on the couch – you've earned it!**

Holding Your Baby

You're going to find yourself carrying the baby around quite a bit during the first few weeks. Babies who are colicky (cry a lot) are often more comfortable if you keep moving, and moving will help reduce your tension and anxiety when you're on hour two of a colic episode. Babies can be held in several ways, and yours may have a definite preference. Some tried-and-tested baby holds include:

- ✔ **Cradle position:** Cradle the baby's head in the crook of your arm. Most people hold the baby on the left side, but go with what works for you.

- ✔ **Over the shoulder:** Some windy babies feel better with pressure on their abdomen, so slinging them up onto your shoulder may help get the wind out. However, spit-up prone babies and vomiters also like this position, so have a muslin square on your shoulder at all times.

- ✔ **Along your arm:** The baby's head rests on your hand looking up, while her body lies on your arm, with her feet pointed at your elbow.

Whichever position you choose to hold your baby in, use it often! Nothing is better for dad and baby bonding than time spent in close proximity.

Co-sleeping Pros and Cons

Co-sleeping, or sleeping with the baby in your bed, goes in and out of fashion. Right now co-sleeping is popular with many parents, although it comes with a twist in some cases: the baby may sleep in a little sidecar, or co-sleeper, that attaches to your bed. You get the whole bed to yourself, but the baby is right next to you.

A traditional Moses basket on a stand also works well, if you're not comfortable sharing the bed with the baby. If you're still debating about keeping the baby in your bed, or even in your room, consider the following advantages:

✔ **Co-sleeping is convenient if your partner is breastfeeding.** Breastfeeding is much easier if you don't have to get out of bed to get the baby.

✔ **You hear the baby as soon as she starts stirring.** While this itself has pros and cons, the benefit is that she doesn't have a chance to work herself into a crying frenzy before a feed.

✔ **It can give you a sense of closeness as a family.** Hearing your baby's soft breathing is reassuring and also enjoyable.

Also consider the following disadvantages:

✔ **Very light sleepers, especially light sleepers with a baby who is also a light sleeper, may find the whole family awake most of the night.** If you're keeping the baby awake, or she's keeping you awake, you're all going to be excessively cranky.

✔ **You may be too worried about rolling over on the baby to enjoy co-sleeping.** If you sleep very soundly, and the baby is right next to you, this can be a concern, but most parents are very aware of the baby's presence. If it worries you, a Moses basket or other sleeping arrangement in the room may be better for you.

✔ **If one of you works odd shifts, you may find getting in or out of the room without waking the baby difficult.**

✔ **When you put the baby in your bed, you eventually have to put her out.** While your child may prefer to stay in your bed until she goes to university, you may want your bed back in a few years' time. Some children don't go quietly into the dark night and put up quite a fight about sleeping in their own rooms.

Remember that even if you don't want the baby in your room with you, baby monitors make it possible to hear the slightest stirring from another room.

Back to Sleep: Helping Baby Sleep Safely and Comfortably

Once upon a time, almost all babies slept on their stomachs. The babies preferred it, they had less wind and if they spit up or vomited they were less likely to choke. Then, in 1992, new recommendations were released about placing babies on their backs rather than stomachs to sleep, claiming that babies were less likely to die of sudden infant death syndrome (SIDS) if they slept on their backs.

A campaign advocating putting babies on their backs went into full swing in 1994, heavily promoted by paediatricians. Within a few years, almost all babies were put to sleep on their backs, at least while they were in the hospital. More than 300 babies still die suddenly and unexpectedly every year in the UK, but ever since parents and carers have been following the risk reduction advice, the number of babies dying has fallen by over 70 per cent.

A baby who is used to sleeping on her back but is placed prone (on her stomach) to sleep, possibly by a caregiver not familiar with the benefits of back sleeping, has an 18-fold increased risk of SIDS.

Side positioning was originally considered a viable alternative to back sleeping, but more recent data suggests that side sleeping also increases the risk of SIDS, as well as the risk of the baby moving from a side to a prone position. To further reduce the risk of injury or death, keep soft fluffy blankets, pillows and bumpers out of the cot, too. A firm sleeping surface is best.

Coping if baby hates being on her back

Many babies truly hate sleeping on their backs. They don't sleep well, their parents don't sleep well and everyone is miserable. What should you do if you and your baby are both desperate to get some sleep?

- ✔ **Tough it out.** Doing so is really hard, but a good night's sleep is not worth the risk of SIDS.

- ✔ **Rock the baby to sleep first.** If she's asleep before you lay her down, she may stay asleep when you place her on her back.

- ✔ **Use a dummy.** Even if you hate them, dummies really do soothe some babies.

Swaddling your little one

Some parents find their babies are calmer and sleep better when they're tightly wrapped in blankets so their arms and legs can't go flying off in every direction whenever they're startled. Nurses swaddle babies in the hospital for this reason (and because it makes them look adorable). Even the most fumble-fingered dad can do this at home, even though it won't look at all like the nurse's version at first. To swaddle, follow these instructions and also refer to Figure 10-1:

1. **Put the blanket on a flat surface like a diamond, with a point up.**

2. **Fold the pointy end at the top down about 6 inches (15cm).**

3. **Put the baby on the blanket, with her head just above the folded-down edge.**

4. **Pull one of the pointy ends on the side across the baby, covering her arms, and tuck it behind her back.**

5. **Bring up the bottom point to the baby's chin.**

6. **Repeat Step 4 using the remaining point of the blanket.**

   Make it tight enough to make the baby feel secure, but not tight enough to cut off her circulation!

Bear in mind that the baby is not going to lay perfectly still during this procedure. It will take you at least a few tries to get it right.

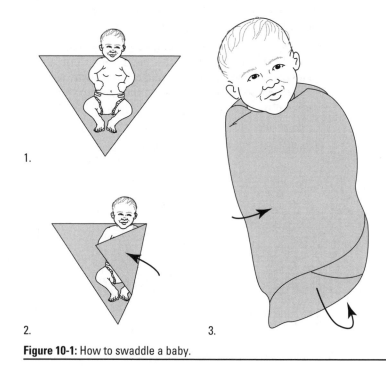

Figure 10-1: How to swaddle a baby.

Preventing the flat head look

Babies now sleep on their backs and also spend hours with their heads back in swings, bouncy seats and car seats. No wonder so many of them have flat heads. A flattened back or side part of the head, called plagiocephaly, can be more than just a cosmetic problem. Though 20 per cent of infants today have flat heads, all but 8 per cent will round out naturally without treatment by 24 months.

You can help prevent plagiocephaly by following these suggestions:

✔ **Have tummy time:** Babies need to spend some time on their stomachs when they're awake to strengthen their neck muscles. This time also gives the back of the head a chance to round out!

✔ **Carry the baby:** Don't always plop the baby in a swing or bouncer when she's awake; carry her around with you so she gets to see more of the world and she doesn't put pressure on her head. Figure 10-2 shows you how to carry your baby in a carrier, if you're interested in doing so.

✔ **Change the room around:** If possible, move the cot from one side of the room to the other from time to time so the baby sleeps with her head turned a different way. Or leave the cot in place and turn the baby, moving her from one end of the cot to the other.

Front pack   Sling   Backpack

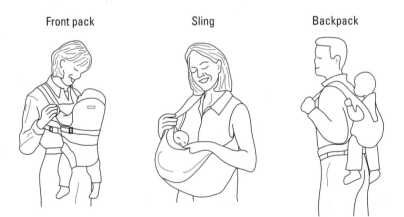

Figure 10-2: A baby carrier lets your baby see more of the world and keeps your hands free in the process.

Plagiocephaly is treated by moulding a custom helmet that exerts pressure on the baby's head and gradually changes the shape as the baby grows. The helmet is worn 23 hours a day and is adjusted as the baby's head begins to round out.

Deciphering cries

Every baby cries a little differently, and every baby has different cries for different occasions. Differentiating the 'I'm hungry' cry from the 'I've got wind' cry or the 'I'm all alone and need company' cry takes practice, but eventually you'll be able to decipher your baby's every need from two rooms away.

And if you have no idea what the baby wants, even when you've had her home for a few months? Do what other parents do: fake it and try everything until something works. Some parents resort to teaching sign language to babies who can't articulate yet so they'll have at least some notion of what she wants. Anything is worth a try.

Having your baby wear a helmet for 23 hours a day for several months is understandably upsetting for parents. It's possible to make helmet wearing more fun – for you, not the baby – by painting the helmet or applying transfers to make it look cute. The babies don't seem to mind wearing them; having the plaster mould of their head done will probably annoy your child far more than the helmet will.

Soothing Baby Indigestion

All babies fuss from time to time, and many have a short fussy period every single day, usually around the time when you're the busiest and have the least patience for it. Although all screaming seems pretty much the same to you, fussiness can be caused by one end or the other of the gastrointestinal tract.

Colic

Colic can send a parent around the bend in no time at all. Colic, defined as three hours of crying a day at least three days a week for three weeks or more in a well-fed, healthy baby, affects around 40 per cent of infants. Colic generally starts between 3 and 6 weeks of age and ends by 3 months of age. They may seem like the longest three months of your life.

No one really knows what causes colic, but colicky babies often pull their legs up to their stomach and act as if they have a tummy ache, so perhaps they do. Breastfed and bottle-fed babies both get colic, and changing the formula rarely helps. Things that help calm a colicky baby include:

- ✔ **Car rides:** The motion of the car calms down many colicky babies. With the price of petrol this can be an expensive solution but, believe us, you'll try anything after the first two hours.

- ✔ **Vibration:** Vibrating chairs or swings calm some colicky babies. If you don't have either of these, you can do what many a desperate parent has tried: putting the baby seat on the dryer and turning it on. Whether it's the motion or the noise, something about it calms some babies. (Stay next to the baby to make sure she doesn't fall off of the dryer!)

- ✔ **Position changes:** Some babies like pressure on their abdomen, so letting her dangle over your arm while you walk around may work. Putting her over your knee, face down, and patting her back may work, too.

- ✔ **Decrease the stimulation:** Some babies don't like being handled or stimulated when they're colicky and do better in a quiet, dark room.

Wind

Babies often need help to get wind out of their stomachs after they eat. Some babies burp it up spontaneously, but others need to be patted between the shoulder blades for a few minutes to get the wind out.

If the baby falls asleep at the end of a feed without burping, don't put her down without getting a burp up. She'll give you just enough time to fall asleep or get involved with something before she wakes up with that piercing cry that means a bubble is stuck. Take a few extra minutes and get her to burp; you'll be glad you did.

Reflux

Although many babies spit up after feeds, gastrointestinal reflux disease (GORD) is a different thing entirely. Gastrointestinal reflux (GOR – not the same thing as GORD), or normal spitting, occurs in over half of all babies, but usually is worse between the ages of 1 and 4 months and disappears by 6 to 12 months.

Keeping the baby in an upright position for half an hour or so after feeds helps reduce GOR, and then keeping her at a 30-degree angle for sleep may help. Some parents elevate one end of the cot to keep the baby's head higher than her feet.

Keeping your cool during baby meltdowns

Babies sense stress, and an already stressed out, screaming baby will be made more unhappy by a stressed out, screaming parent. To help maintain control in difficult situations, try these ideas:

✔ **Leave the house:** You and your partner can take turns getting out of the war zone for a short time.

✔ **Close the door:** For periods of time when you can't leave the house but truly can't take it anymore, put the baby in her room and close the door for a few minutes.

✔ **Get help:** When a crying baby brings you to the brink, you may be shocked at how quickly your anger escalates. Anger management courses can help you tame an out-of-control temper. Learning to do it now rather than later is beneficial, because this child will be doing things to drive you crazy for the next 50 years. (No, parenthood isn't easier when your children are adults!)

Despite what you may be told, studies show that thickening the formula with cereal does not help, and it may worsen respiratory problems in children with GORD.

GOR is annoying and potentially ruinous to your clothing and the baby's, but GORD is a more serious problem. Babies with GORD fail to gain weight, may have respiratory difficulties from milk aspiration and may have feeding aversion, which is understandable since food so often brings them discomfort.

Breastfed babies are less likely to develop GOR or GORD, because breast milk digests more easily and empties out of the stomach twice as fast as formula. Medications to reduce stomach acid or to keep stomach acid from entering the oesophagus may be prescribed to treat GORD.

Scheduling Immunisations

Immunisations are a very hot topic today, and one that many parents have vehement opinions about. Although studies have not supported fears that immunisations are responsible for the increase in children diagnosed with some forms of autism – a neural disorder characterised by impaired social interaction and communication skills – many parents believe there is a link.

Marking the milestones

Baby books are a wonderful invention; it's a shame more parents don't use them throughout their child's infancy. Most parents start out with great enthusiasm, recording every pregnancy symptom, movement and ultrasound. But when the actual baby arrives, time is precious and the baby book is often neglected, although an occasional guilt trip may result in copious recording for a week or so.

Make every attempt to record your baby's milestones somewhere. You don't have to use a baby book; baby calendars, your own journal or a blog can be used to keep track of your baby's first tooth, word or step. You may think now that you could never forget such important milestones, but the sad truth is that you can, very easily. And if you have more than one child, trying to remember who had croup and who had chicken pox gets to be impossible. And when you have grandchildren, many years from now, you can prove to their parents how much more advanced the grandchildren are compared to them at the same age!

The number of injections a baby receives in her first year can seem overwhelming. Table 10-1 shows the average newborn schedule of immunisations (some of the series are continued after the first birthday).

Table 10-1   Average First-Year Immunisation Schedule

Vaccine	2 Months	3 Months	4 Months	1 Year
Diphtheria/Tetanus/ Pertussis	x	x	x	
Haemophilus influenzae type B	x	x	x	x
Pneumococcal	x		x	x
Inactivated Poliovirus	x		x	
Meningitis C		x		x
Measles/Mumps/ Rubella				x

Skipping some injections?

Immunisations are so controversial in some circles today that you may consider giving the baby some but not all of the recommended vaccines, possibly skipping influenza, hepatitis and chicken pox vaccines and splitting the measles-mumps-rubella injection into three separate injections. Talk seriously with your doctor about the advisability of splitting the vaccines in this way – almost all will say don't do it!

Spreading them out

Many parents compromise on the immunisation question by spacing the vaccines over a longer time period than recommended. Taking more time may necessitate more visits to the doctor than are normally scheduled but can make it easier to determine which injection is causing a reaction if a problem occurs.

Chapter 11

Supporting the New Mum

. . . .

. . . .

A new baby is a celebrity, with every coo, smile and gurgle met with a flash of the camera. A doting parent or grandparent is always ready to meet baby's every whim, and your protective nature makes you feel like you could uproot a tree if it somehow threatened the well-being of your baby. Unfortunately, that limelight is taken away from the woman who just spent the better part of a year carrying that child and hours (or days!) in labour. She suddenly goes from living as an A-list celebrity to feeling like an out-of-work actress.

This is your chance to step up and shine, new dad, by making sure your partner feels every bit as adored, pampered and attended to as that new bundle of joy. This means taking care of tangible needs, like making sure the cat's litter tray is clean and dinner's on the table, and also less-tangible needs, like emotionally supporting your partner, limiting guests and getting by on less sleep.

We know that the upheaval of a new baby can be a difficult adjustment for new dads, too, but rising to these challenges has long-term benefits for the health and happiness of your whole family. The following sections help guide you through the postnatal needs of your partner and show you how to be a hero for the new mum in your life.

Handling Housework during Recovery

New mums and dads both experience the stress of adapting to a new little person who's still a stranger to you, but mums have the added burden of uncontrolled hormones and physical recovery from the delivery. Your partner's energy needs to be directed at keeping herself together right now, not worrying about the house – or you.

While your partner recovers, gets her hormones back together and settles into her new routine as a mum, she needs you to pick up the donkey work around the house without being told what to do. You may not know exactly what that entails, but that's why we're here: to help you with all the things that need to be done. The following sections may look like a list of chores, but remember that a happy mum means a happy baby – and a happy next six months for your new family.

Getting the house in order

If you believed the adverts, men are only good for making messes and women derive joy from cleaning up after them, but in the real world, making sure the home is in tip-top shape is everyone's job. Except that now that your partner's limited to lifting nothing heavier than a baby for the next six weeks, cleaning has just become fully your responsibility.

You don't have time to clean every part of the house every day, so ask your partner point-blank what tasks are most important to her; then carry out her requests word for word – even if they seem irrational. For example, if she wants the bathroom cleaned every day, then grab your toilet brush and get scrubbing. She'll be spending a lot more time in there following labour because of postnatal bleeding, which can last anywhere from two to eight weeks, so a clean environment may help her relax and keep her from feeling embarrassed when visitors unexpectedly appear.

Speaking of visitors, well-wishers come bearing a lot of stuff, which means that clutter can get out of control very quickly. Because mum is trapped indoors with a baby who's feeding around the clock, feeling suffocated by balloons, flowers and stuffed animals may only increase her anxiety. Make sure to find a new home for everything that comes into the house.

In addition, doing the dishes, hoovering and taking out the rubbish are some of the obvious tasks that need regular attention. The following sections guide you through some of the more unexpected tasks you're about to become intimately acquainted with.

Battling baby's bottomless laundry basket

Laundry may seem straightforward, but like all things related to babies, it's complicated. If you're already accustomed to the ins and outs of laundry, you'll have ample opportunity over the next few weeks to put these basic skills into action. But laundering baby's things is a bit different. We break down the important points for you here:

- ✔ **Wash brand-new infant clothes prior to first use to remove any chemicals or germs in the fabric.** As new clothes arrive, be sure to remove all price tags, stickers and plastic tag holders.

- ✔ **To avoid exposing your baby to dyes and chemicals that can irritate his delicate skin, wash baby clothes in dye- and chemical-free washing powder.** Generally, any washing powders labelled as dye- and chemical-free are okay to use. Using organic is always best but can be quite pricey. Several washing powders, such as Dreft, are designed specifically to wash baby clothes.

- ✔ **Use the delicate cycles on your washer and dryer.** Using the delicate cycle helps keep the materials used in baby clothing from shrinking, which they tend to do. And baby clothes are outgrown fast enough without adding shrinkage to the mix.

- ✔ **Be sure to treat stains – and you'll have stains – prior to washing.** Spray on or rub in a stain removal product before putting the garments in the washing machine.

Couples opting to take the eco-friendly route of cloth nappies find the mounting laundry pile an even taller task. Follow these steps to take care of this particularly dirty laundry:

1. **Rinse the nappies.**

   Solid poo can be shaken off into the toilet and flushed. Consider installing a sprayer attachment on your toilet to help with loose stools and urine. It allows you to rinse the nappies and flush without having to dunk the nappy into the toilet.

2. **Pretreat cloth nappies by sprinkling stains with bicarbonate of soda (you'll find it in the baking section at the supermarket) and then soaking them in a bucket of hot water.**

   Buy a bucket with a lid to keep the smells at bay. You can also place an air freshener inside the bucket as an extra precaution.

3. **Gather a load of no more than two dozen nappies, fastening all tabs on each nappy to keep them from sticking to each other.**

4. **Use a quarter to half the amount of washing powder you'd use for a normal load.**

   Using a normal amount can lead to detergent build-up in the fabric. Nappies are designed to absorb, after all, and they're not discriminating about it.

5. **Wash on a cold/cold cycle.**

6. **Wash a second time, using a hot/cold cycle to kill any remaining bacteria.**

Dealing with pet duty

Animals require a delicate transition when the baby arrives. To help reduce the shock of a new human roommate, prior to bringing baby home from the hospital, wash your pet's bed or favourite toys in baby washing powder to get him used to what baby will smell like. You can also prepare your pets by inviting over friends with babies so your animals become familiar with the sounds they make.

No matter how well trained or prepared your pets are, take care when introducing your baby. When baby comes through the door, be prepared to deal with any jumping, clawing, growling or playing your pet may want to engage in with both mum and baby. Keep animals separated from mum until she's healed enough to endure any unexpected pet reactions. When you trust that your pet won't react wildly, have the animal sit next to you while you hold the baby. Reward your pet with treats as you interact with the baby to begin making a positive connection between the two. Never hold your baby in your pet's face as doing so can prompt a possibly dangerous reaction from the animal.

In addition to mediating interactions between your partner and rambunctious pets and baby and *all* pets, it's also your responsibility to complete all pet-related tasks. That means changing the cat litter, taking the dog for walks, grooming and playing. Making sure your pet's life stays as normal as possible eases everyone's transition. For example, if your dog enjoys playing catch, try to play catch with him as often as you did before so he doesn't make a negative association between the new baby and your lack of attention.

After contact with your pets, make sure to wash your hands with soap and water before handling the baby.

Becoming the errand boy

Grab the keys and get rolling, because driving duties are up to you for a while. Doctors recommend that women who have a vaginal birth don't drive for two weeks following delivery. That time increases to six weeks for a caesarean delivery.

The weight game

Your partner may not be ready to get back into her pre-pregnancy jeans the moment she gets home from the hospital. Some women do lose a considerable amount of weight shortly after delivery, but some actually put on weight as a result of fluid retention. And as with all weight loss, unfortunately, losing pounds put on during and after pregnancy requires time and hard work.

Exercise helps the body recover from pregnancy (and has also been linked to decreased occurrence of depression), but even with exercise, it takes an average of two or three months before a woman gets back to her normal body weight. And even then, things will have changed. Stomachs are softer, body parts seemingly have shifted, stretch marks will have appeared, and she's likely to feel like a stranger in her own body.

You can help your partner improve her body image and fitness by reminding her how beautiful you think she is and planning activities that get you both moving together. A nice walk around the park or the neighbourhood is always an enjoyable activity for the whole family, and following a normal childbirth, women can begin light walking a few days after returning home. If the gym is her scene, ask her if she'd like you to hire a personal trainer with knowledge of post-pregnancy fitness. If the yoga studio is her style, she may enjoy a mum-and-baby yoga class.

Whatever her desires, make sure she's been cleared by her doctor or midwife prior to beginning any workout routine, and she'll likely be advised to stick with activities that she engaged in before having the baby. She needs to start small, and you need to make sure your partner is comfortable. Remind her to exercise at a slow pace with moderate effort, especially during the first weeks. If she experiences an increase in bleeding, shortness of breath or extreme fatigue, persuade her to wait a few days before trying again.

Most importantly, let any new exercise regimen be her idea. Suggesting that a new mum should join a gym will put you squarely in the doghouse.

Use the hours you spend driving to the shops and the post office (to mail thank-you notes, of course!) to recharge your batteries. Alone time is hard to come by these days.

Don't forget to extend an invitation to mum and baby, too. Many women will begin to feel trapped in the house, so as soon as your partner is up for it, begin including her in outings whenever she wants to come. If she doesn't feel up to it or can't come along for the ride, bring her back some flowers or another favourite treat to make her feel loved and cared for.

Taking care of meals

For the first few weeks following delivery, you need to manage the meals, because your partner is probably too physically drained – and too busy feeding baby – to think about cooking. Whether you're the guy who likes to take charge in the kitchen or the type who routinely forgets to add the cheese to macaroni cheese, making sure you and your partner are well nourished is one of your most important roles.

Understanding what she needs

Breastfeeding women need to consume an additional 400 to 600 calories more than they would when eating a normal diet. That's because breastfeeding burns about as many calories as a 30-minute run. New mums need to eat energy-packed, nutritious foods. And with all the extra work you're doing on reduced sleep, you do too! Keep the following nutrition do's and don'ts in mind when out shopping and preparing meals:

- ✔ **Do** stock up on milk, yoghurt and other dairy products. Vitamin D and calcium are especially important for new mums. Some women are forced to eliminate dairy from their diets because it can cause excess wind and fussiness in the nursing baby. In order to get her the nutrients she otherwise would get from dairy, stock-up on plant-based milk substitutes, such as soya or almond milk, which have been fortified with vitamins.

- ✔ **Don't** bring home a lot of foods that are high in sugar, carbohydrates and fat. Nothing is forbidden here, but don't go overboard. Not only is it bad for her waistline, but all the refined sugars, flours and artificial fats are hard to digest and aren't ideal postnatal nutrition for baby or mum. As hard as it is to deny a new mother anything, try to talk her out of those cravings for fried food.

- ✔ **Do** make sure she's getting enough water. If she's breastfeeding, she needs to drink at least two litres of water each day to aid in milk production. If your tap water doesn't taste good, pick up a filtration jug or tap attachment.

✔ **Don't** let her (or you!) drink too much alcohol. A glass of wine or a beer is okay, especially as a way for the new mum to clear her head and relax. But nursing mums should keep in mind that what goes in ends up in the breast milk, so moderation is essential. Non-nursing mums, and dads for that matter, still must be responsible caregivers, and alcohol lowers inhibitions and decreases sound judgement. Always drink very responsibly.

In addition to taking her nutritional requirements into account, make sure to ask her what sounds good before doing any food shopping. Just like during pregnancy, many women find certain foods unappetising and/or nauseating following childbirth.

Putting food on the table

Since you're going to be getting less sleep and doing more work around the house, you may not be eager to strap on the apron three times a day. To make the task easier on yourself, cook meals that can be eaten multiple times or frozen for future consumption, such as easy-to-assemble casseroles or pots of soup. If time allows, this can be a great nesting activity with your partner prior to delivery, too.

Another great idea that only requires a little work on your part is to make a batch of sandwiches, put them back in the bread bag, and store the bag in the fridge, so that she can just grab one quickly. This would be especially helpful for a mum who's going to be home alone during the day when making good eating choices may be next to impossible with a baby whose needs come first.

Make sure mum has plenty of nutritious foods around that she can just grab and eat without either of you having to prepare them. Yoghurt, nuts, fruit and precut, precleaned raw vegetables should be on hand as quick energy boosts that require no cooking.

When friends and family ask you what they can do to help, ask them to bring you a meal in a freezer-safe storage container in lieu of flowers. Having prepared homemade meals to hand will help you avoid the temptation to order takeaway or fast food, which is high in sodium and fat and not the most nutritious for mum and baby.

Calling in back-up

Not every new dad has the luxury of taking ample time off work to attend to the needs of his partner, which means your partner may be facing a lot of alone time with baby at a very early stage.

Leaving a new mum alone while you're off at work isn't a good idea. Many women, especially those who delivered via caesarean section, need physical and emotional support during the daytime for several weeks following delivery.

Talk to your partner about the needs and desires she has while you're at work, then help her find the appropriate support from friends, family and neighbours. Make chore lists for daytime helpers so your partner won't feel embarrassed by having to ask for help.

If financially viable, employ a cleaner. Doing so will be the best gift you can give to your partner . . . and yourself.

Following the birth of their grandchild, your parents and partner's parents may want to visit during this time in order to help, especially when you go back to work. Before agreeing to visits, however, make sure your partner wants them around. All of the advice and constant companionship from a parental figure may cause her more stress. She also may want a chance to go it alone without anyone's help.

If she does want them around, try to stagger the visits to provide a longer duration of coverage – and a little more sanity for you and your partner.

Supporting a Breastfeeding Mum

Breastfeeding is a full-time job, especially in the first few months, and although it may be more fun and rewarding than changing poo-filled nappies, it's still a lot of responsibility. To the untrained eye, it may look like your partner is simply sitting in a rocking chair holding your baby, but she's actually working very hard to develop a complicated feeding relationship. This section shows you how you can help mum and baby be as successful as possible.

If you feel really lost on this subject, check out *Breastfeeding For Dummies* (Wiley) for more in-depth encouragement.

Making the decision to breastfeed

If your partner is physically capable of breastfeeding (some medical conditions prevent women from doing so), the decision is ultimately hers. It's her body, her time and her commitment. Prior to the arrival of baby, discuss this topic so that you can both research the benefits of breastfeeding and decide whether or not to do it and, if so, for how long.

Breastfeeding is an important health choice, and any amount of time a mother and baby can do so benefits both. Breastfeeding is a natural process, and the milk contains disease-fighting cells that help protect infants from germs, illness and even SIDS (sudden infant death syndrome – turn to Chapter 12 for more info). Infant formula, while meeting the requirements of basic nutrition, does not include the human cells, hormones or antibodies that fight disease.

For the new mother, breastfeeding is a wonderful bonding experience that has been shown to decrease the risk of postnatal depression and lessen its impact. It also causes more afterpains, which are spasms that help shrink the uterus back down to normal size. Producing milk also burns anywhere from 200 to 500 calories a day. Studies also show it reduces a woman's risk of breast cancer and increases her bone density after baby is weaned, reducing her chances of developing osteoporosis in the future.

The health benefits for baby and mum are good reasons to breastfeed, but be sure your partner considers the following details when making the decision:

- ✔ **Convenience:** Breastfeeding is much more convenient at home than bottle-feeding, but it can be awkward when you're out and about. Although many shopping centres, museums and amusements parks have mother and baby rooms, not all do, and your partner may not be comfortable nursing in public. That's why supplemental bottles were invented.

- ✔ **Comfort:** Some women are not comfortable with the idea of breastfeeding. Don't blame your partner. This discomfort may arise from a culture that makes breasts into sex objects rather than feeding machinery.

- ✔ **Ability:** Breastfeeding isn't possible following breast reconstruction surgery that cuts the milk ducts.

- ✔ **Schedule:** If your partner is going back to work in a few weeks, establishing nursing may seem like too much trouble. But nursing for even a short time is better than not nursing at all. Encourage her to try, for even a short time. Just don't be pushy about it.

Many specialists recommend breastfeeding for the first year of a child's life, and the World Health Organization recommends breastfeeding for the first two years. However, the benefits of breastfeeding continue for as long as mother and baby do it, whether it be three days or three years. The more you support your partner in breastfeeding, the more unparalleled health benefits your baby will receive.

Whether you start off baby with formula or switch after a period of breastfeeding, do your research about the best, safest formula for your child. Many breastfed babies resist the transition, so be patient. Then again, you're probably used to that by now.

Offering lactation support

If your partner chooses to breastfeed, keep in mind that it's not as easy as it looks, especially at first. Issues will arise, and although you can't be the one to solve those issues, your support is a major factor in her success. Be positive and upbeat, listen to your partner when she talks and thank her profusely for making such a wise decision for both the baby's health and hers.

The most important role for dad is to stay informed about the process of breastfeeding. Many complications can arise, and the more you know about how to help your partner through those issues, the more likely mum and baby will be able to work through them. One of the most common reasons women have for ceasing breastfeeding is that it is uncomfortable or painful. Breastfeeding *should not hurt* after mum and baby establish the correct feeding and latching on (how baby attaches his mouth to the nipple) positions.

Some of the most common breastfeeding issues are

- ✔ **Sore nipples:** This problem is usually temporary during the first few days as mum adjusts to breastfeeding. For some women the pain increases, and the nipples become chapped or cracked. This is most commonly the result of poor latching on and can be treated by correcting how the baby attaches his mouth.

- ✔ **Pain from breast engorgement:** Engorgement occurs when the breasts fill up with milk, and can be eased by massage, milk expression and warm compresses.

- ✔ **Clogged ducts:** This occurs when the breast has not been completely emptied and it becomes clogged, causing a small lump to form inside the breast. Heat packs, massage and increased feeding from the clogged breast can treat it.

- ✔ **Mastitis:** Mastitis is a breast infection that a small percentage of breastfeeding women get. It can cause flu-like symptoms and a hard lump in the breast. Treat with warm compresses, painkillers and a trip to the doctor for a course of antibiotics.

Breastfeeding 999

If your partner is experiencing discomfort or suffering from a low milk supply, know where to go to get her the help she needs. Potential sources if your partner needs breastfeeding guidance include:

The Association of Breastfeeding Mothers: www.abm.me.uk

The Breastfeeding Network: www.breastfeedingnetwork.org.uk

La Leche League GB: www.laleche.org.uk

The National Childbirth Trust: nct.org.uk

Remember that it's the mother's decision to quit breastfeeding if she so chooses and should never be your suggestion. If lactation issues arise, don't tell her to throw in the towel and buy some formula, no matter how frustrated or tearful she becomes. Listen to her concerns, help her find resources to correct problems and, ultimately, be supportive no matter what she decides.

Whenever your partner decides for any reason to stop breastfeeding, thank her for the time she's invested in doing so and congratulate her for her achievements. You should both be proud of the hard, rewarding work you've done.

Including yourself in the process

Just because mum does the actual breastfeeding doesn't mean that you can't be involved, too. An important role for you is to serve as your partner's arms and legs while she breastfeeds, especially in the early stages while your partner's mobility is severely limited by a baby who eats at frequent intervals all day long. Let your partner know that you're happy to get her anything she needs and thank her for breastfeeding the baby. The more you can anticipate her needs, the better. Always have a drink and snack at hand, as well as the TV remote and something to read.

Many women feel frustrated by not being able to do things for themselves. Reassure your partner that baby's constant eating schedule is only temporary and that it won't be long before he eats less often and her mobility returns. Until then, make sure to bring your partner everything she asks for without hesitation.

Sometimes fathers of breastfed babies feel as though they're missing out on an important, unparalleled bonding opportunity. Remember that breastfeeding is about the well-being of your child, and although you can't ever experience what your partner does, you can join in on the skin-to-skin bonding by letting baby rest on your bare chest. You can also occasionally give baby supplemental bottles of pumped milk. (See Chapter 10 for more on supplemental bottles.)

Dealing with Post-Caesarean Issues

Not only is the hospital stay longer following a caesarean section than a vaginal delivery – two to four days total – but the recovery time upon returning home is extended as well. A caesarean delivery is classified as major surgery, which means that even if everything goes smoothly, you have to care for a woman who has been through nine months of pregnancy followed by a serious operation. You will also need to be on the lookout to make sure that no complications arise while your partner is recovering.

Helping with a normal recovery

Give your partner additional physical support for the first few weeks. She shouldn't engage in vigorous exercise or household chores or even climb a lot of steps. If you have to go back to work during the first two weeks post-delivery, find a family member or friend who can come to your home and provide all-day support for your partner.

Emotionally, it's important for the new mum to sit and bond with her baby following a caesarean. Some women experience feelings of disappointment and can even struggle to bond with a newborn when unable to give birth vaginally. Most, however, have no trouble bonding after spending some time together.

If the operation was unexpected, many new dads and mums need some time to debrief following the stress of the situation. Following the birth, discuss the events leading up to the caesarean with your partner. Some new parents find it helpful to discuss the events with the obstetrician to help deal with any negative feelings they have about their birth experience.

Pain management is important following a caesarean, and when not properly managed it can reduce the chances of successful breastfeeding and increase the risk of postnatal depression.

Encourage your partner to ask her doctor about appropriate pain-relief medication and how it will affect her breast milk.

Knowing when to call the doctor

Most women who deliver via caesarean recover quickly and without incident. However, watch out for these warning signs and contact a doctor immediately if your partner

- ✔ Has a temperature over 100 degrees F (37.8 °C).

- ✔ Notices pus leaking from the incision.

- ✔ Suffers a swollen, red, painful area in the leg or the breast, possibly accompanied by flu-like symptoms.

- ✔ Complains of a painful headache that does not subside.

- ✔ Experiences abrupt pain in the abdomen, including abnormal tenderness or burning.

- ✔ Has a foul-smelling vaginal discharge.

- ✔ Experiences an unusual amount of heavy bleeding that soaks a sanitary towel within an hour.

- ✔ Feels abnormally anxious, panicky and/or depressed.

Riding the Ups and Downs of Hormones

If feeling physically well while exhausted and still carrying a few pounds of extra baby weight wasn't hard enough for a new mum, along come the hormones to make it all even worse. As the body recovers from childbirth, several months are needed for a woman's hormone levels to completely even out. This section overviews the many changes your partner may experience and how to deal with them.

Thinking before speaking in the sensitive postnatal period

If you've ever put your foot in your mouth, then you know that you can accidentally hurt your partner's feelings as a result of your own thoughtlessness. After delivery you need to be even more careful of what you say, because for most new dads, your partner's emotional sensitivity will feel like uncharted shark-infested waters.

Avoid using leading statements, such as 'why don't you just' and 'why didn't you' when your partner is upset. You don't have all the answers, and she's not looking for answers, anyway. What she's probably seeking is a listening ear and an understanding hug. The last thing you want to tell a tearful new mother when she confesses to feelings of isolation is, 'Why didn't you just go out today?' She's probably worked very hard all day taking care of herself and the baby, and flippantly suggesting that she should have done more than she did can make her feel like a failure.

To show support, ask her questions that show you're listening, such as 'What would make you feel better?' and 'What can I do to help you?' If your partner responds with 'I don't know' or 'Nothing will help until the baby is older/sleeps more/cries less', then tell her you want to help in any way possible. If she has trouble expressing what she needs, you may find yourself becoming frustrated with your inability to fix the problem. Until she can express her needs, plan some time for her that doesn't force her to make any decisions but instead pampers and caters to her needs and shows her how much you care.

When your partner is upset about something you said, bear in mind that hormones are at play, but don't suggest to her that hormones are the reason she's being sensitive. The last thing you want to do is imply that her feelings aren't legitimate. Simply apologise for any and all offending statements and let her know that you understand where she's coming from.

Many new mums also become sensitive to anything involving hurt or neglected children, which can make TV programmes, films and books potential minefields. To the best of your ability, research the contents of your entertainment. If the film you want to watch involves a child death, botched childbirth, kidnapping or the destruction of the Earth, put it on your to-do list for later viewing.

Shedding light on physical symptoms

Body-drenching night sweats are very common for new mums, and you can't do much to help except set up a fan near the bed. Sudden hair loss is another physical effect of surging hormones. In the first few months following delivery, most women begin to notice a lot more hair coming out in the shower and on the hairbrush. Reassure your partner that this hair loss is normal and that it usually goes back to normal by nine months after delivery. If it doesn't, help her seek treatment from a dermatologist.

Supporting her baby blues

Happiness is only one of the complex emotions you and your partner will feel following baby's arrival. The most common and complicated issue for new mothers is the baby blues, feelings of exhaustion, insomnia, irritability, nervousness, panic and that she'll never be a good mother, which usually occurs during the first few weeks following delivery. Studies show that nearly 80 per cent of women suffer feelings of sadness and loss post-delivery.

Experts believe that shifting hormone levels are partly to blame but that it's also difficult for a woman who has been focused on giving birth for nine months to suddenly switch gears and focus on nurturing a newborn. Caring for a child stirs strong emotions and can make new parents feel an overwhelming sense of responsibility and fear, both of which are perfectly normal.

Talk openly with your partner about her feelings, as well as any sad feelings you may be experiencing. Keep reading to find out how to determine if her baby blues are something more serious that needs treatment.

Recognising postnatal depression

While most new mothers experience some feelings of sadness that eventually pass, 10 to 15 per cent of all new mothers suffer from depression during the first six months post-delivery, and depression requires some care and treatment. Distinguishing between the baby blues and postnatal depression is not as difficult as you may think, especially for you. Your partner may not be able to put her feelings into words or admit she's depressed, but you can be alert for signs of depression and have a discussion with her if you recognise any symptoms. Common symptoms include

- Lack of interest in caring for self or baby.
- Loss of appetite.
- Relentless unhappiness.
- Incapable of being happy while spending time with baby.
- Sudden arrival of anxiety and panic attacks.
- Hearing voices.
- Disturbing thoughts about harming self or baby.

If you believe your partner is depressed, tell her that you're concerned about her health, allow her to discuss her symptoms and
how she's feeling, and let her know that what she's dealing with is
a serious medical condition. It doesn't mean she's a bad mother or
a weak person. Good and strong people can suffer from postnatal
depression. Don't let her brush the issue aside by saying that it's
just a matter of feeling sad and that she'll snap out of it, because
she won't.

A depressed new mum needs to be treated by a medical professional immediately, so work with your partner to schedule a session with her doctor. Counselling and antidepressants are very
effective treatments.

Sleeping (Or Doing Without)

Surprise! It's a baby who doesn't sleep through the night.
Depending on your newborn, you may be woken every hour on the
hour for feeds and comforting. Or you may be one of the lucky parents catching hours and hours of uninterrupted sleep. Every baby
is different, but one thing is constant: sleep is a precious commodity for new parents.

Babies' sleeping habits change frequently, but the average newborn
sleeps about eight hours during the day, waking up every hour or
so to eat. They generally sleep another eight hours during the night,
again waking frequently to eat. Newborn sleep cycles are shorter
than those of adults, and they spend more time in light sleep than
adults do, which accounts for the frequent disturbances.

The common rule is to sleep when your baby sleeps. A million
chores may need to be done around the house, and you may enjoy
an hour watching tennis in peace, but close your eyes instead. If
you nap during the day when you have a chance, you'll be in much
better shape to deal with a baby who's ready to party when you're
ready for pillow time at night. You can take turns with your partner
throughout the night, alternating who gets up each time or switch-
ing nights. Use a schedule that works for you both.

Many babies wake up for good before the sun has a chance to hit
the horizon. If you're routinely jarred from sleep at an obscenely
early hour, alternate days of getting up early with your partner so
at least one of you can get some additional sleep. That way, when
the early riser's energy wanes later in the day, the other partner
can step up to help out.

A baby's internal sleep clock begins to mature between the ages of 6 and 9 weeks and starts to become constant between 3 and 5 months. By 10 months, the average baby's sleep cycle is constant, and he will go to bed and wake up at the same time every day. If you're still awake by that time and haven't become addicted to caffeine, congratulations. Your sleep cycle will start getting longer, too.

Many babies begin sleeping through the night at between 4 and 6 months. Then again, many babies begin sleeping through the night at 1 year of age. Both are normal. Consult your doctor if your baby's sleep pattern is unmanageable for you and your partner.

Coping with Company

Family and friends will be vying for any opportunity to get their hands on your baby. Being surrounded by love is important at this time, but mum, dad and baby also need to get plenty of rest and to have sufficient time to bond as a family. And getting plenty of rest and private family time will help keep you from lashing out at your mother when she offers yet another helpful pointer about the proper way to fold bath towels.

Try not to schedule multiple visitors at a time, and limit the number of visits to two or three per day. Now is also the time in your life when it's okay to cancel or say no to visits. If Aunt Sarah is scheduled to drop by in the evening and your partner just needs to catch some shut-eye, put your partner's needs first. Reassure Aunt Sarah that she will get to see the baby in due time. If she's offended, she'll get over it the moment she holds your baby for the first time.

You and your partner should decide together when it's a good time to have people over and when you need some peace and quiet. However, your partner may feel guilty about saying no even when you know very well that having an empty house is in all of your best interests. Don't be afraid to turn people away without asking your partner so she doesn't always have to feel like the bad guy.

As visitors cycle through your home, make sure they all wash their hands or use an alcohol-free hand sanitiser to avoid spreading germs. If someone is unwell, it's your duty to keep him out of your home. Thank him for his support but let him know that exposing newborns to illness is dangerous.

Baby will be passed around a lot when company is visiting and often only handed back to the new mum for feeding. Make sure that your partner gets plenty of non-feeding time with the baby to avoid having her feel like a dairy.

Dealing with grabby grandmas

Sharing isn't easy – especially for new grandmas. And as they will gladly tell you (again and again), someday you'll understand when you have a grandchild of your own. Until then, you need to manage everyone's needs for the next 20-plus years without offending anyone.

The best way to handle a too hands-on grandma is to be honest and respectful. If you want to hold your baby and your mother or mother-in-law is reluctant to hand him over, reach for the baby and say something like, 'I just can't hold this little one enough. I've been waiting for this moment my whole life.' There's nothing like a display of paternal love to remind a grabby grandma how important bonding is between parent and child.

Don't be passive-aggressive in your approach. Avoid asking questions like, 'Mum, do you think I could hold the baby now?' You don't want to imply you think grandma is being overbearing, thoughtless or disrespectful of your time.

If the problem persists, speak to the offending parent in private. Thank grandma for her love and support, and use only *I* statements (such as, 'I have really been feeling the need to spend more time bonding with my baby right now, and even though it may not be what everyone would want, I really need this time') to convey how much you want to spend time with your baby.

Managing unsolicited advice

One of the first things to raise the ire of a new parent is a pushy, well-meaning advice giver. Everyone seems to have opinions when it comes to how to care for your baby, and if you start paying attention to everyone, it will completely overwhelm you. So just run. Run far, far away and don't look back.

Whether the advice is on how to hold him, how to burp him or even how to soothe him when he's having a crying session, try to internalise the fact that most people are reaching out with advice because of the love they feel for your newborn. When advice comes across as criticism of your parenting skills, shrug it off. You and your partner know your baby's needs and preferences better than anyone else. Defer to your instincts. Every baby is different, and what works for one may not work for another.

Of course, you may find some advice helpful, so be open to listening to what others who have parented before you have learned. Don't be afraid to reach out to others if you have questions, but never take someone's advice as gospel. Take the time to do your own homework and decide what works best for your family.

Don't feel the need to explain yourself, however. If your Uncle Robert thinks you're somehow failing your child by picking him up every time he cries, don't be afraid to push back. Say something like, 'I guess the beauty of being a parent is getting to decide how you want to raise your own child.'

Handling hurt feelings when you want to be alone

Inevitably at some point you'll need time to yourself. So will your partner. Baby love is all encompassing, but you can't let it overtake your individuality. Even though visitors have travelled from afar and people want to shower your new family with affection, you still have to find time for yourself. Whether you're a runner or an avid computer gamer, don't feel guilty about taking time to do what you need to relax.

Never under any circumstances utter the phrase, 'I just need a break'. Your partner won't want to hear that, because nobody deserves a break more than a new mum. Let her know that you really need to blow off some steam in order to continue being the best caregiver you can be. If she's angry, tell her you understand how she feels and offer her the same amount of time upon your return. Even the breastfeeding mum can enjoy a brief walk or a quick run to the shops just to have some time to be on her own again.

Make sure to schedule time for your mental well-being, because it probably won't seem like a priority until you're raving like a madman because you just need a second of solitude. Keep a calendar and block out times in different colours for family time, dad time, mum time and visiting hours.

If family or friends take offence when you say no to a visit or an invitation to attend a family function, don't change your mind to save their feelings. You deserve time to bond as a family and time to unwind and just be yourself. Thank them for the offer, be honest about why you can't commit to that time and plan a get-together for a later date that suits everyone's schedule.

Approaching Sex: It's Like Riding a Bicycle

Hang tight, fellas. It's going to be a while. The earliest a woman can usually have (or want!) sex is six weeks following delivery. Your hormones may be raging, but you need to remember that your partner's genitalia have been through the wringer, so to speak, and intercourse can severely jeopardise her healing process.

In addition to needing time for physical healing, most women won't be feeling all that sexy for a while. Hormones are the major culprits, but lack of sleep, breastfeeding and the difficulty of strad-dling the roles of mother and sexual being are also hurdles. As hard as it is to internalise, remind yourself that her lack of physical interest in you has nothing to do with her feelings toward you. Her absence of desire isn't personal; it's physical.

Some women find their sexual desires return by the time their doctor okays sex, but for many it can take between 6 and 12 months. Some new fathers also experience a diminished interest in sex when adjusting to the role of dad.

Even after your partner has healed and desire returns, she may experience discomfort when returning to a normal sex life. Be pre-pared to take it slowly. You may need several attempts before you actually have sex to completion. Time is also an issue and baby may wake up before you finish.

Time will also be at a premium as you work around baby's sched-ule, so as unromantic as it sounds, schedule sex with your partner and slowly ramp up to a frequency that works for both of you. With so much on your plates, it will give you both the security of knowing the 'when' and the excitement of thinking about the 'how'.

Birth control also needs to be a talking point for you and your partner. Many people believe that breastfeeding women cannot get pregnant, but although breastfeeding does often delay a return to regular ovulation, some women do ovulate while nursing. Many breastfeeding women prefer not to go on the pill, so condom usage is common for new parents returning to active sex lives. You can speak with a doctor to help you both determine a birth control option that fits your needs.

Part IV
A Dad's Guide to Worrying

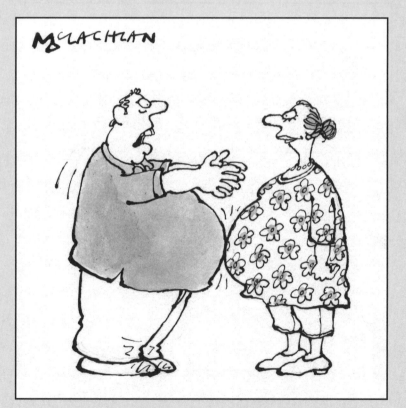

"Don't let the baby come between us, Fiona."

In this part...

This part is designed to keep you from staying up all night worrying about all the things new dads worry about, from colic to college. We discuss possible complications and newborn concerns, and we devote a whole chapter to being a supportive partner, lest you forget the person who gave birth to your progeny. We also help you plan for your child's future financial security.

Chapter 12

Dealing with Difficult Issues after Delivery

*N*ot everyone goes home to perpetual roses and lollipops after their baby is born. In fact, hardly anyone does. But serious issues in baby or mum are rare, so when they occur, they can really knock you for six. In this chapter we discuss some of the serious complications that can arise after delivery and how to handle them. This is a chapter you can skip if you don't need it – and we hope you never will.

Coping with Serious Health Problems

The latest figures from the Office for National Statistics show that, in England and Wales, 62 in every 10,000 live or stillbirths have some degree of congenital anomaly. Developmental delays, serious illnesses and sudden infant death syndrome are problems no one wants to contemplate when having a baby, but they can and do happen. The following sections give you an overview of the most common serious health problems.

Congenital defects

Congenital defects, defects that exist at birth (also simply called *birth defects*), are common. Some are minor issues that no one but the parents would ever notice; others are more serious. The most common birth defects include

- ✔ **Heart defects:** One in 145 babies born in the UK has a congenital heart defect, ranging from very mild to severe. Heart defects comprise one-quarter to one-third of all birth defects.

- ✔ **Down's syndrome:** One in 1,000 babies born in the UK has Down's syndrome, which causes distinct physical features and mental retardation. The percentage is higher in older mothers and lower in those younger than 35.

- ✔ **Neural tube defects:** Just over one in 1,000 infants born in the UK has neural tube defects, which affect the brain and spinal column. They include spina bifida, an abnormal opening in the spine, and anencephaly, an absence of part of the brain.

- ✔ **Cleft lip and/or palate:** One in 700 babies in the UK has deformities of the lip and hard palate.

Sixty per cent of the time, the reason for the birth defect is unknown. Inherited disorders, on the other hand, may be suspected ahead of time if a family history of a genetic disorder exists.

Some of the most common inherited genetic disorders include

- ✔ **Cystic fibrosis:** A disorder that causes thick secretions in the respiratory and gastrointestinal tract, cystic fibrosis is the most common inherited genetic disorder in Caucasians in the UK, affecting five babies born every week. Both parents must carry the defective gene for a child to have the disease; it's estimated that 2 million people in the UK are carriers.

- ✔ **Sickle cell anaemia:** An autosomal recessive disease causing deformities of the red blood cells, sickle cell anaemia affects mostly people of African and Middle Eastern descent. Approximately one baby in every 2,000 in the UK is born with this condition.

Minor birth defects are much more common than serious defects. Eye, ear and limb defects; extra digits; abnormal development of the intestines; and birthmarks may not be life threatening in most cases, but they can still be devastating for parents. Being concerned about birth defects, especially visible ones, is normal for parents.

Developmental delays

Many parents keep baby books that chronicle their baby's progress, and eagerly await each milestone: the first smile, the first step, the first word. When milestones aren't met when books say they should be, or when your friends' babies are meeting them but your baby isn't, doubt, concern, frustration and a cold fear may begin to creep into your days.

 Mums are usually the first ones to recognise a problem, so if your partner voices concerns, don't belittle them, even if the baby seems fine to you. Verbalising fears about your baby's development takes a lot of courage.

When babies are very young, physical milestones are very important. Babies, after all, don't dazzle you with their small talk or charm you with their recitation of *The Iliad*. If they lift up their head, it's a big deal. Rolling over for the first time merits phone calls to relatives all over the country, and the first gurgle – the one that startles the baby almost as much as it does you – earns your undivided attention for the next hour as you try to catch a command performance on video.

When your baby isn't keeping up with the other babies on the block (whether in your mind or in fact), discuss it with your doctor, who may tell you that all babies are different and that you're making yourself crazy. Or she may nod and take notes, which is really frightening, because even when you know something's wrong, having someone else verify it makes it all too real.

If you suspect that your baby isn't meeting developmental milestones, take a deep breath and consider the following facts:

- ✔ **Babies really do develop at different rates.** Milestones happen at an average age, and an average is just that: 50 per cent of babies achieve the goal at a younger age, and 50 per cent don't meet it until they're past that age.

- ✔ **Babies all have different abilities.** Some are more physically orientated; others are more verbally inclined. Since physical milestones are all you have to go on at a young age, children who will shine verbally later may seem to be behind early on.

Talk to your doctor if your baby doesn't meet the following milestones:

- ✔ Turns her head in the direction of a voice or sound shortly after birth.

- ✔ Smiles spontaneously by 1 month.

✔ Imitates speech sounds by 3 to 6 months.

✔ Babbles by 4 to 8 months.

If your baby does experience developmental delays, she'll need your help to achieve normal milestones. Getting help early is the best thing you can do for her.

Illnesses

Infant illness can be *acute* (severe but brief) or *chronic* (long lasting or recurring). Both are terrifying, especially if your baby has to be hospitalised. An ill baby, especially a chronically ill baby, changes your family dynamic in major ways and can become the unhealthy focus of the entire family. The following suggestions can help you deal with an illness in your infant, whether acute or chronic:

✔ **Absolutely, positively avoid any hint of the 'blame game'.** Even if anything either of you did caused the baby to become ill, it's over and done with, so pinning blame on someone will only make everyone feel worse. Babies can't be raised in a bubble, so getting ill is, unfortunately, a fact of life.

✔ **Don't let yourselves get overtired.** Especially if your partner delivered not too long ago, she really needs to get enough rest. Take turns staying at the hospital or being up with the baby at home, or one of you could get ill, too.

✔ **If your partner is breastfeeding, keep pumping.** Stress is hard on milk supply, and pumping isn't nearly as effective as a nursing baby for stimulating the supply, but encourage your partner to do her best. As long as she keeps it going in the interim, the supply will build up when the baby is breastfeeding again.

SIDS

Sudden infant death syndrome, or SIDS, has decreased since paediatricians began recommending that babies sleep on their backs, but it's still the third most common cause of death for infants up to one year old. More than 300 babies in the UK succumb to SIDS each year.

Identifying the causes and debunking myths

The causes of SIDS still are not clear. However, doctors know that the following are *not* causes of SIDS:

✔ Suffocation.

✔ Choking.

> ✔ Vomiting.
>
> ✔ Infections.
>
> ✔ Immunisations.

SIDS is considered to be multifactorial, meaning that it doesn't have just one cause. Several factors must all be present for SIDS to occur, including abnormalities in the brain, respiratory system and possibly the heart.

Understanding what increases the risks

The following factors increase the likelihood of SIDS:

> ✔ The baby was born prematurely.
>
> ✔ The baby is male.
>
> ✔ The baby is black.
>
> ✔ The baby is between 2 and 3 months of age.
>
> ✔ The baby is overheated or overdressed. Too many clothes or an overly heated room may increase the risk of SIDS. SIDS occurs more often in cooler autumn and winter weather when babies get bundled up.
>
> ✔ The baby has a sibling who died of SIDS.
>
> ✔ The baby was/is exposed to tobacco. SIDS rates are higher in babies whose mums smoked during pregnancy or who smoke around the baby.
>
> ✔ The mother used cocaine, heroin or methadone during pregnancy.
>
> ✔ The baby recently had a respiratory infection.
>
> ✔ The baby sleeps on her stomach, especially if she's switched from back to stomach sleeping or is overheated and sleeping on her stomach.

Research also indicates that babies who are breastfed and those who suck on dummies may have a lower risk of SIDS. Side sleeping may seem like a compromise if your baby hates being on her back, but back sleeping is still safer, and many side sleepers roll over onto their stomachs.

Placing a fan in the window, or even just opening a window, also has been shown to decrease the risk of SIDS in at least one study. SIDS deaths dropped more than 70 per cent when a fan was placed in a window and dropped 36 per cent when the window was opened. Better ventilation may decrease carbon dioxide build-up.

Watching Out for Postnatal Issues

Female hormones are a jumbled mess right after delivery, which is why women are so emotionally fragile after birth. Add sleep deprivation and insecurities about parenting ability, and it's amazing that your partner can function at all.

Mood swings and depression are normal for the first few weeks or even months after having a baby, but sometimes more serious problems can arise. One of your jobs is being aware of the signs of a serious problem and making sure your partner gets help if needed.

Getting through the 'baby blues'

Nearly every new mum experiences the 'baby blues', emotional mood swings and mild depression triggered by hormone changes after delivery. Symptoms of baby blues include

- ✓ Anxiety or feelings that she's not doing things 'right'.
- ✓ Crying for no reason – at least, for what seems like no reason to you.
- ✓ Difficulty concentrating.
- ✓ Irritability.
- ✓ Mood swings.
- ✓ Periods of sadness.
- ✓ Trouble sleeping.

Baby blues normally last just a few weeks after giving birth, so if symptoms last longer or seem more severe, get your partner to her doctor for help. Many women don't recognise the severity of their own symptoms or don't have the emotional energy to deal with them.

Taking a look at postnatal depression

Postnatal depression, a more serious form of the typical baby blues, occurs in up to 10 per cent of women. Some of the symptoms of baby blues and postnatal depression overlap, but postnatal depression is more pronounced, lasts longer and includes serious signs that need immediate medical evaluation.

Recognising the symptoms

Women with postnatal depression may have the following symptoms:

- ✓ **Difficulty bonding with the baby:** This is a major red flag. If your partner pushes the baby off on you or says she's not a good mum or that the baby would be better off without her, get medical help.

- ✓ **Thoughts about harming herself or the baby:** She may not verbalise these thoughts, so they may be hard to recognise. She may want other people to handle the baby because of her fears that she'll hurt her, accidentally or on purpose.

- ✓ **Guilt and shame over her negative thoughts:** Again, because she may not verbalise her thoughts, recognising what's going on may be difficult. Statements like 'I'm no good' or 'Someone else would be a better mum to this baby' are warning signs.

- ✓ **Sleep difficulties:** She may not be able to sleep, or she may want to do nothing but sleep.

- ✓ **Disinterest in normal activities, including sex:** Seeing old friends, going out, even everyday activities like cleaning the house, doing laundry and watching TV may all go out of the window. While you may at first think she's just tired, a deeper reason may be at the root of her continued lack of interest in life that lasts for several months after delivery.

- ✓ **Loss of appetite:** Losing interest in eating is often an early sign of depression.

- ✓ **Anger and irritability:** Her anger may go far beyond a few swear words when she drops a glass, and can be frightening.

Postnatal depression usually is not a short-lived disorder, so don't try to wait it out, thinking she'll get over it in a week or two. Postnatal depression can last up to a year, which can interfere with maternal–child bonding and seriously disrupt your family.

Children of mums with untreated depression also suffer the consequences, and present a higher incidence of behaviour problems, sleeping disorders, feeding problems, hyperactivity and language delays.

Knowing who's more at risk

Any woman can have postnatal depression, but the chances of this developing increase if

✔ **She has a history of depression.**

✔ **She's recently undergone major life changes.** These changes can include a move, a death, job loss, illness, pregnancy complications or trouble between the two of you.

✔ **She doesn't have a good support system.** Family and friends make a big difference in the life of a new mum. Postnatal depression makes it difficult to reach out to others, so a woman who doesn't have pushy friends and family who will check in on her even if she doesn't call them is very isolated.

✔ **The pregnancy was unplanned or unwanted.**

Treating the disease

Treatment for postnatal depression may include

✔ **Antidepressants:** Make sure the doctor knows if your partner is breastfeeding so an antidepressant safe for use by breast-feeding mums can be prescribed.

✔ **Hormone therapy:** Oestrogen replacement to offset the rapid drop in oestrogen after giving birth may be helpful for some women.

✔ **Counselling:** Talking things out with a professional is very helpful for some women.

Taking care of yourself

If your partner is suffering from postnatal depression, a large part of her normal chores and responsibilities may fall on you. If you're trying to hold down a job, make sure your partner's okay, make sure the baby's okay and run the household on top of it all, you may start to feel a little stressed yourself.

While rushing in to take over a short-lived crisis is easy, a situation that drags on for months can take its toll on your mental and physical well-being. Take care of yourself by making sure you

✔ **Get enough sleep.** Sleep deprivation makes everything look worse. The very worst time to pore over your worries is the middle of the night; everything seems insurmountable at 3 a.m.

✔ **Eat properly.** You'll feel better and be better able to handle situations if you're not eating junk food.

✔ **Call in the troops to help.** You may not have readily available family and friends, but if you do, enlist their aid. Send them to the shops, or have them come over and clean. This is a fine line, because you don't want to give your partner the impression that she can't do all this stuff, even when she can't. If you call in your mum to clean or cook, your partner may view it as a judgement against her abilities and a sign that you feel your mum is more capable than she is. Sometimes hiring help for household chores is a better idea.

Acting fast to treat postnatal psychosis

Postnatal psychosis is an extremely dangerous psychiatric disorder that occurs in around 1 to 2 per cent of women, usually in the first few weeks after giving birth. Women with bipolar disease or a previous history of postnatal psychosis are more likely to develop the condition. Onset is sudden and includes the following symptoms:

- ✔ Paranoia.

- ✔ Hallucinations.

- ✔ Delusions.

- ✔ Insomnia.

- ✔ Irritability.

- ✔ Restlessness.

- ✔ Rapidly changing moods.

- ✔ Bizarre thinking.

Left untreated, postnatal psychosis can be lethal; the risk of suicide or infanticide is high. If your partner displays any of these symptoms, don't try to talk her out of it or persuade her to see her doctor. She almost certainly won't recognise her behaviour as abnormal and in fact will probably consider you to be an adversary. Call 999 immediately.

Managing Grief

Grief is intense sorrow as the result of loss. The loss of the perfect child, the perfect partner or perfect family can cause grief. The most important thing to remember about grief, no matter what the cause, is that it takes time to work through. Don't be hard on yourself or your partner when you're grieving, and don't expect you'll be in the same stages at the same time. Everyone works through grief differently.

Going through the stages of grief

Grief can be caused by many different scenarios, but the widely acknowledged five stages of grief, described by psychiatrist Elisabeth Kübler-Ross, include similar phases whatever the cause.

Whether you've found out that your baby has a long-term problem, your partner is suffering from serious postnatal illness or your baby has to be hospitalised, expect to experience the five stages of grief:

1. **Denial:** The first stage of grief is often a feeling of 'This can't be happening to us'.

2. **Anger:** The second stage of grief is anger, often directed at God or other people.

3. **Bargaining:** Trying to make secret deals – 'I'll donate our savings to this hospital if my baby's heart surgery saves her' – often with God (even if you don't believe in God!) is common in the bargaining stage.

4. **Depression:** When reality sets in and you realise that this is happening to you, fair or not, depression often follows.

5. **Acceptance:** Eventually you get through the other stages and settle down to dealing with what you have to deal with, but you may still go in and out of earlier grief stages at different times.

Stages may not follow this exact pattern, and not everyone goes through every stage. Yo-yoing back and forth between several stages is also common.

Why, why, why? Getting past the question

When grieving, getting bogged down in why a particular thing has happened to your partner or child is easy to do. However, dwelling on the reason isn't particularly good for you, especially if there's no way of deciphering exactly why something happened and most of your thoughts are purely speculative.

Unless knowing the reason why your problem happened can prevent a recurrence or change a situation, asking 'why' doesn't help. Wanting a reason is a way of imposing control on a situation, but it doesn't help you move forward in helping your child.

Grieving together and separately

Everyone needs time to grieve a loss in their own way. Grieve together with your partner, certainly, but take time to grieve separately as well. Don't feel bad about needing to be alone with your thoughts sometimes. At the same time, the following tips can help you and your partner get through your grief, both together and on your own:

- ✔ **Stay physically close.** It helps you feel less alone, keeps you centred on still being a couple and helps keep your relationship going in a situation that could easily break it apart. Even if you don't feel like it, make the effort to hold hands, cuddle on the couch watching TV and have sex regularly.

- ✔ **Expect to be discouraged at times.** Everyone has moments when things look much worse than they really are, usually because they're tired, hungry or just plain stressed. Identify it for what it is: temporary discouragement, not a new permanent negative outlook on life.

- ✔ **Don't get upset with your partner.** One day you or your partner may be raging against the world, and the next day the other one may take a turn. Listen to each other without taking things personally, trying to make it all better or reproving them for their feelings.

- ✔ **Arm yourself with knowledge.** Knowledge really is power. Especially if your baby has a genetic or long-term condition, learning all you can about it helps you be your baby's best advocate and can help you and your partner feel like you're doing something productive in a frustratingly out-of-control situation.

- ✔ **Keep a journal, if the thought appeals to you.** Journals are not only good for privately venting feelings and fears that you and your partner don't want to share with each other; they're also good for looking back later and realising how far you really have come.

- ✔ **Find a support group.** If you're coming to terms with a birth defect, your child or partner is ill or you're dealing with a loss, talking to other parents dealing with the same thing can be a lifesaver. When relevant, it can also be a really good source of information on specialists, educational programmes and other outside help.

- ✔ **Get help for yourself.** If you find yourself mentally overwhelmed, seek counselling, either with your partner or alone. Often just being able to talk through a situation with a person not involved helps you sort things out.

✔ **Tell people when you're not up to something.** Another baby's christening, a big family party or a holiday celebration may all be beyond your or your partner's ability to handle at first. Don't be afraid to say no to things that you feel would strip you raw right now. People who love you will understand, even if they're disappointed.

Determining when grief has gone on for too long

Grieving can take a long time. But sometimes grief takes on a life of its own, and a situation called *complicated grief* can become permanently entrenched in your or your partner's life. While everyone has times when the sadness of circumstances becomes overwhelming, normally these feelings don't affect every aspect of life after the first few weeks or months. Complicated grief may be taking over your life or your partner's after a period of time if

✔ You still feel numb and detached.

✔ You're preoccupied and bitter about what's happened.

✔ You can't perform normal tasks, go to work or participate in normal social functions.

✔ You feel life has lost its meaning.

✔ You're unusually angry, irritable or agitated most of the time.

✔ You make rash decisions or do things you normally wouldn't do, such as drinking too much.

Talking through change

Even if your baby is born without incident, you will be going through a lot of changes. Allow yourself and your partner to discuss the many things you're giving up in order to bring this child into the world.

Even something as silly as giving up your daily latte in order to buy nappies can become a source of resentment over time. As a general rule, talk openly and honestly about the changes that affect you and support each other.

And give yourself a break – parenting isn't easy, and it's perfectly natural to miss having nights out with friends or even being able to eat an entire meal before it gets cold. Grieving over the little things doesn't mean you don't love your baby – it means you're dealing with change in a healthy manner.

When grief becomes complicated, it becomes self-perpetuating. This is a time for intervention, either with medication or therapy. Talk to a grief counsellor, psychologist, psychiatrist or other mental health professional about your feelings and symptoms. Antidepressants have been found to help in some cases.

Talking to Other People about Your Child

Accepting a child's health problems is challenging enough for parents, and an emotionally sensitive situation is made even more difficult by the fact that eventually you need to inform other people of the problem. In time you may become accustomed to the comments of well-meaning but blundering family members and rude strangers, but at first you will likely be uncomfortable and upset. The following sections give you guidelines for getting through these situations.

Telling other people

Telling other people that your child has a problem can be gut-wrenching; verbalising to other people can be almost like hearing it for the first time yourself. When you tell other people your child has a problem, try the following tips:

- ✔ **Keep it simple.** Especially if your child has an ongoing medical problem, giving out information a little at a time may make it easier for others to digest.

- ✔ **Keep it positive.** Maybe your child isn't going to be able to be all you ever hoped for her. Actually, no child ever can! Remember that your child will be able to have a happy life, no matter what her disability, and you can enjoy her no matter what her issues. That positive outlook will express itself in your message.

- ✔ **Keep it straightforward.** You may be tempted to sugarcoat a situation when explaining it to others, but there's no reason to give them hope that a child will grow to be something she won't. Be honest about the situation from the beginning.

Handling insensitive remarks

Unfortunately, people do notice when a child has a birth defect or is developmentally delayed and sometimes you hear them whispering to each other or pointing at your child. As devastating as this is, use it as a teaching experience if you can. If your child has a visible birth defect, comments *are* going to come your way – and your child will hear and understand those comments as she gets older.

Openly discussing your child's disability as something not to be hidden or ashamed of sets a positive example for your child. This doesn't mean that you have to freely discuss your child with every obnoxious person who asks pointed questions. But addressing questions with an open, accepting, positive attitude tells your child – and everyone else – that she's a great kid and that you're happy with her just the way she is.

Sometimes you won't have the patience to deal with questions, and you don't have to educate every person who crosses your path. But when your mood allows it, try the following suggestions when confronted with insensitive remarks:

- ✔ **Answer a small child's questions.** Children, having no discretion at all, often ask their parents about people with visible problems. Introduce yourself and use this opportunity to teach others about your child's disability.

- ✔ **Address an adult's comments in a non-judgemental way, if you're up to it.** Most insensitive remarks are made out of ignorance, not malice, and even if they were made out of malice, addressing them politely can take the wind out of a person's sails and, with any luck, shame them into better behaviour in the future.

- ✔ **When your own relatives are saying inappropriate things, address the situation firmly and in a non-negotiable way.** Offer to teach them anything they'd like to know, but let them know in no uncertain terms that this is your child and certain comments will not be tolerated.

Chapter 13

Daddy 999: Survival Tips for Bumps, Lumps and Scary Moments

· ·

In This Chapter

▶ Surviving the illnesses and accidents

▶ Staying cool and handling emergencies

▶ Giving medicine, taking temperatures and monitoring nappies

▶ Helping your child through teething

▶ Taking a look at reactions to vaccines, medications and food

· ·

*N*othing in fatherhood gets your adrenaline flowing like a thump from the other room, followed by a scream, or worse, by silence. Nothing, that is, except endless vomiting, fits or a shunt while you have baby in the car.

Fatherhood is full of frightening moments, but most of the time babies survive parental ineptitude. No one gets through babyhood and early childhood without a few accidents, sicknesses and spills and thrills along the way. If your child never has a bruise or bump, you're probably protecting him too much, and a child who never gets ill never develops a good immune system. So take heart when dealing with heart-stopping situations: they're an inevitable part of parenthood. In this chapter we review the most common sources of parental anxiety, tell you what to do when they occur and reassure you that, 99 times out of 100, baby – and you – will be just fine.

Breastfeeding when mum is ill

Mums aren't allowed to be unwell – it says so in the parenthood code. But if your partner does become ill while breastfeeding, you may both wonder about the wisdom of continuing to breastfeed.

If she's already ill, the baby's already been exposed to the germs before the illness became evident, so no reason exists for her to avoid the baby. Very few illnesses require her to stop breastfeeding. In fact, mums who develop colds and other common illnesses develop antibodies that they pass on through the breast milk, so nursing when ill may actually help the baby. Toxins such as E. coli, salmonella, botulism and other gastrointestinal bugs stay in the GI tract and don't affect the milk, so breastfeeding is safe.

Your partner should check with the doctor if she's taking heavy-duty cold medication that has a sedative effect, and she should avoid cough syrups with alcohol contents over 20 per cent. Nasal sprays for sinus congestion can dry up her milk, so use sparingly.

When your partner is ill, she's likely to require higher than usual amounts of fluid to stay hydrated – and a double dose of TLC to keep her going through night-time nursing sessions. Getting up yourself and giving a bottle of pumped breast milk for a night or two so she can sleep will buy you bonus points as a helpful dad.

Handling Inevitable Illnesses

Most babies are now vaccinated against the most common illnesses, but plenty of illnesses can still infect your baby. And no matter how hard you try to protect your baby from illness-causing germs, you can't protect him from them all – and that's okay. Although hand washing, careful food handling and cleanliness do help reduce germs, some germs are necessary. In fact, recent studies indicate that people who keep their homes too bacteria-free are more likely to become unwell than people who share their abode with a few stray germs. Explain that, if you can.

You can be sure that your baby will catch something in his first year, no matter how carefully you clean the shopping trolley handles. In the following sections we describe the symptoms, causes and treatments of common illnesses so you'll feel prepared when the inevitable happens.

Nursing baby through common childhood diseases

Babies have immunity to many illnesses for their first six months because of antibodies passed on during pregnancy, but after six months, it's open season for germs. Following is a rundown on the most likely candidates for first illness to infect the baby.

Common colds

The common cold is so common that it comes in more than 100 varieties, which is why having a cold this month doesn't mean you won't get another one next month. And because your baby has never had any of them, he's likely to have at least one case of the sniffles in the first year. In fact, the average baby has eight to ten colds in the first two years of life, and each one lasts seven to ten days, no matter how many decongestants you buy. You may want to consider stocking up on tissues!

For most babies, colds aren't serious, although they are messy. Typical symptoms of a cold include:

- Runny nose, which may start with clear, thin secretions that become thicker and yellow or green.

- Sneezing.

- Coughing.

- Decreased appetite (young babies may find it hard to breast-feed or drink from a bottle because of nasal stuffiness).

- Low-grade temperature (under 100.4 °F/38 °C).

- Irritability.

Babies under the age of 3 months should not be given decongestants at all, and infants younger than 6 months should be given them only if congestion interferes with breathing or sleeping. Infant paracetamol is recommended if below 3 months, and paracetamol and ibuprofen if older than this.

Ear infections

Between 5 and 15 per cent of babies with colds develop an ear infection, which just prolongs the misery. Contrary to popular opinion, tugging on the ears doesn't always indicate an ear infection, although it can. Other ear infection symptoms include:

✓ Irritability

✓ Head shaking

✓ Refusal to breastfeed or take a bottle

✓ Mild temperature

✓ Trouble sleeping

The thinking on treating ear infections has changed during the last few years; ear infections may not require antibiotic treatment, because more than eight out of ten heal without treatment. Some doctors treat, and others wait, depending on the severity of the infection and the symptoms. Pain relievers help with discomfort.

Respiratory syncytial virus (RSV)

Respiratory syncytial virus (RSV) is a lower respiratory illness that infects most children at least once before age 2. Symptoms include lethargy, poor feeding, cough, difficulty breathing and a temperature. While most cases are mild, severe illness requiring hospitalisation can occur in small babies and premature or otherwise compromised infants.

For less severe cases, which occur far more frequently, paracetamol or ibuprofen help with discomfort. Like most viruses, this one just needs to run its course.

Vomiting

Small children and babies vomit more easily than adults when they're ill. Vomiting once at the beginning of an illness is common and requires no special treatment, but repeated vomiting requires medical evaluation because of the risk of dehydration.

Serious dehydration requires medical treatment. A sunken *fontanelle*, the soft spot on the top of an infant's head, extreme lethargy, sunken eyes or sunken skin that remains raised after you pinch it deserve an immediate call to your doctor.

Paediatricians often recommend giving vomiting children younger than 6 months an oral balanced-electrolyte solution such as Dioralyte in place of formula, starting with a few teaspoons or half an ounce every 15 minutes or so. Don't give plain water to any child younger than age 1 unless your GP specifically recommends it. A medication syringe often works better than a spoon if your baby refuses to drink. Gradually increase the amount you give each time if the baby isn't vomiting it back up.

Don't give a volume more than you normally would: for example, if you normally give 4 ounces of formula every four hours, don't exceed that amount.

If no vomiting occurs after 12 hours, slowly start to reintroduce formula, but stop if vomiting occurs again. Breastfed babies should continue to breastfeed, because breast milk is more digestible than anything on the planet. However, if vomiting continues, call your doctor.

Babies who suddenly start vomiting after every feed even though they appear healthy and still have an appetite may have *pyloric stenosis*, a narrowing between the stomach and small intestine. Pyloric stenosis requires surgery but has no after-effects; when it's fixed, it's fixed. However, the baby may have something more common than this – gastro-oesophageal reflux. This can also cause vomiting after feeds and does not require surgery, usually just some medication . . . and they usually grow out of it!

Wheezing

Wheezing often follows a cold and doesn't always mean a baby is going to have asthma. Children younger than age 2 who wheeze with respiratory infections are no more likely to develop asthma than children who don't wheeze. In contrast, children who start wheezing at an older age are more likely to develop asthma.

Wheezing can be scary for parents, and may require prescription bronchodilators that are breathed in as a mist, using a nebuliser, to open the narrowed airways and make it easier for the baby to breathe. Wheezing requires a call to your doctor, especially if the baby doesn't have a cold or cold symptoms. An object stuck in the throat or more serious medical conditions can also cause wheezing. Some children wheeze with every upper respiratory illness and may need nebuliser treatments whenever they have bad colds.

A child who is limp and exhausted, who has a bluish tinge around the lips or who is struggling to breathe needs immediate medical attention.

Infectious diseases

Many infectious diseases of old (30 years ago!) have been eradicated, or nearly so, as a result of vaccines (see the 'Reacting to Medicines and Vaccines' section later in this chapter). However, vaccines haven't been developed for everything, and sometimes a baby is exposed to an infectious disease before he gets the vaccine. Vaccines for chicken pox, measles, mumps and rubella (German measles), for example, aren't given until age 1, and roseola, a common infectious disease in infants, has no vaccine.

Being viruses, most common childhood diseases have no specific treatment beyond treating the symptoms and keeping the child comfortable. Aspirin should never be given to treat a temperature or discomfort, because of the possibility of a connection between the potentially fatal Reye's syndrome and aspirin consumption by children with viral illness. Ibuprofen is fine if your child is uncomfortable; follow your doctor's instructions on dosing – and infant paracetamol is fine.

Many infectious diseases are accompanied by rashes, so any time your child has a rash and a temperature, call your doctor for advice. He may want to see your child, but then again, in some cases, he may not want you bringing your infectious child into the waiting room! If the disease is highly contagious and fairly evident from the type of rash, such as chicken pox, he may give instructions over the phone without seeing the child. Following are some common infectious diseases with rashes:

- **Roseola:** Roseola has few complications but often results in frantic calls to the doctor because the first symptom, which lasts for several days, is a high temperature. Around day four the fever breaks and a rash appears. A telltale sign of roseola is that even with a temperature as high as 102.2 °F (39 °C), the child doesn't appear ill. Roseola has no treatment and generally doesn't cause a great deal of discomfort.

- **Chicken pox:** Chicken pox is unmistakable – small red spots that form blisters that break and crust. A mild temperature and respiratory symptoms often accompany chicken pox. In rare cases, chicken pox can cause encephalitis – brain inflammation that can have long-term consequences. There's no way to shorten the duration of the disease, but cool baths and anti-itch lotions (such as calamine lotion) help with discomfort.

- **Hand, foot and mouth disease:** Although this sounds like some ghastly disease only vets would catch, hand, foot and mouth disease is a common virus that causes blisters on the – yes, you guessed it – hands and feet and in the mouth. A mild temperature can also occur, and the mouth sores can make it hard for a child to eat.

- **Measles:** Also called rubeola, measles was once a common disease, but the number of cases fell to fewer than 400 in 2010. This decline is attributable to the MMR vaccine. Measles rarely occurs before age 6 months because of maternal immunity being passed to the foetus. Children with measles usually appear quite ill and have a rash and a high temperature.

- **Rubella:** Rubella, sometimes called German measles, is a mild infection that causes a rash. While not serious for infected children, rubella poses serious risks for pregnant women, causing a number of birth defects, including blindness, as well as pregnancy loss. Rubella has become rare in the UK as a result of vaccination.

> ✔ **Mumps:** Mumps causes pain and swelling in the parotid glands, resulting in the classic 'chipmunk' appearance. Mumps, like measles and rubella, has become rare in the UK because of the mumps vaccine. Mumps can cause painful testicular infection in males but results in sterility less than previously believed.

Staying alert for scarier diseases

Some heavy duty bacteria and viruses can infect infants, but the signs are usually pretty obvious: your baby looks and acts unwell, refuses to eat, cries and sleeps too little or too much. Rest assured that if your baby is seriously ill, you'll recognise the signs. In the following sections we tell you what to watch for.

Meningitis

Meningitis, an inflammation of the tissues that cover the brain, can require hospitalisation. Meningitis can be bacterial or viral and is caused by a number of organisms. Vaccination for *Haemophilus influenzae* type B, also known as Hib, reduces the chance of meningitis. Symptoms include a high temperature, irritability, poor feeding, a rash, seizures, a high-pitched cry and a stiff neck. In infants, the soft spot at the top of the head, the fontanelle, may be bulging rather than flat. Signs of meningitis mean your child needs immediate treatment to prevent complications.

Diarrhoea

Although diarrhoea may seem like more of a nuisance than a serious disease, severe diarrhoea can cause life-threatening dehydration in an infant within a day or two. Diarrhoea accompanied by a temperature, vomiting or refusal to drink fluids needs immediate treatment. Diarrhoea is most often caused by bacterial or viral illnesses, including food poisoning.

The following symptoms indicate serious dehydration that needs a doctor's treatment:

> ✔ Extreme lethargy.

> ✔ Sunken fontanelle (the soft spot on top of baby's head).

> ✔ Sunken eyes.

> ✔ Sunken skin that remains raised after you pinch it.

Loose, frequent stools aren't always diarrhoea; see the 'Deciphering Nappy Contents' section later in this chapter for ways to distinguish diarrhoea from normal stools.

Protecting Baby from Common Accidents and What to Do When They Happen

You may not think newborns have a lot of accidents, since they're not all that mobile, but they do. In this section we go over the most likely scenarios and tell you how to handle them.

Taking care of baby after a fall

Even a newborn can shift himself enough to fall off the changing table or bed, which is why you're not supposed to leave a baby unattended, without your hand on him, for even a second. Babies usually bounce pretty well and rarely break bones in a fall, but the parental guilt may be enough to put you in a rest home for a week.

Even worse is the 'I was holding the baby on the couch and the next thing I knew there was a thump' fall. Most common in the first sleep-deprived weeks of parenthood, the 'I dropped the baby' fall devastates guilty parents. Avoid the guilt by not lying down on the couch holding the baby – and don't sit up holding him if you're feeling really sleepy, either.

Parents rarely drop babies when they're walking, but a trip on the pavement or over a misplaced toy can send you and baby sprawling. Whenever the baby goes to ground, watch for these signs that a medical evaluation is in order:

- ✔ **Prolonged crying:** Every baby cries after a fall, if for no other reason than that landing on the ground is startling. Besides, you're crying, so baby thinks he should be, too. However, crying that lasts more than a few minutes may indicate an injury that should be checked out.

- ✔ **No crying:** Obviously, if your baby is completely unresponsive after a fall, call 999 immediately. Give him a minute, though; he may be too stunned to cry for a few seconds.

- ✔ **Repeated vomiting:** A baby who falls with a full stomach may spit up, but repeated vomiting can indicate a head injury.

- ✔ **Sleepiness:** This is one of the trickiest judgement calls of parenthood: what do you do when the baby falls just before bedtime? Keeping a tired baby awake is nearly impossible, and you shouldn't wake him up every few minutes just to make sure he's still responsive. Watch him for an hour and keep him awake if possible, but don't stress if it's not. If it's naptime or the middle of the night, let him sleep, but assess his breathing and colour for any changes every few hours and watch to make sure he's moving normally in his sleep. Breathing that becomes very heavy or deep may indicate a problem.

✔ **Inability to move a body part:** Babies' bones are still made of mostly cartilage, which bends easily, so he's unlikely to break a bone in a fall. If a mobile baby refuses to crawl or use an extremity, have it checked out.

✔ **Gaping cuts:** If he falls on a metal object and comes up bleeding, see if the wound's edges are close together or gaping. Gaping wounds usually need stitches, glue (no, this is not a do-it-yourself project!) or butterfly stitches. Take your baby to a doctor or hospital.

✔ **Huge bruises:** Foreheads are famous for developing immense bruises after a bump. Bruises alone aren't concerning, unless they're accompanied by other signs, such as sleepiness, or if they keep growing. Bruises that bleed excessively can be a sign of other diseases, such as haemophilia, and need to be evaluated.

Staying safe in the car

Car accidents are a fact of life, and you can't always prevent other drivers from driving badly or from running into your rear end at a red light. This is why a properly fitted, age-appropriate, approved car seat is absolutely essential.

A newborn should never, never, never be held in a moving vehicle. Not in the front seat, the back seat or anywhere else. Numerous studies have proven you cannot hold on to an infant in an accident; the baby will fly out of your arms and straight out of the front or side window into the street, or will be tossed around the car like a rag doll.

Yes, this warning is meant to create a vivid picture that will scare you into never travelling in a car with your child in your arms. Babies die this way every year because they were taken out of the car seat to be fed or soothed for a moment. A moment is all it takes.

The following is essential car-safety information for your baby:

✔ **Put newborns and small infants in a car seat designed for their weight.** Never put a newborn in a seat designed for an older child, or vice versa.

✔ **Never put infants and small children in the front seat, even if they're in an approved car seat.** The front seat is much more dangerous for your child if you're in an accident. Getting your baby in and out of the car is easier in the front seat, but put him in the back. Please.

✔ **Use rear-facing car seats for infants up to at least 12 months and 20 pounds (9 kg) at a minimum.** Riding facing backwards is safer in the event of a crash, and paediatricians now recommend keeping children rear facing up to the weight limit of the seat they're in. Children don't mind riding backwards, even up to age 2 or longer, and you can place a mirror so you can see them.

✔ **Don't use a car seat beyond its expiration date.** Yes, car seats have expiration dates, usually on a sticker on the side of the seat. The plastic can degrade over time, making the seat unstable in a crash.

✔ **Don't re-use a car seat that has been in an accident.** The car seat may have been weakened or damaged in the accident and may not perform as expected if you have another accident. Getting a new one is worth the extra money.

✔ **Don't borrow a car seat unless you know the expiration date and know it's never been in an accident.** Don't take chances on a car seat that may be damaged in any way, even if it looks fine.

✔ **Read the instructions so that you install the seat correctly.** A huge percentage of car seats are found to be incorrectly installed when checked at car seat clinics.

✔ **Don't carry dangerous loose items, like shovels in the car.** They become missiles in an accident.

If you're in an accident, check the baby carefully for bruises and cuts, especially if the car seat is dented or banged up at all. Remove the car seat from the car with the baby in it if you can so you can check for signs of injury without causing more injury to the neck or back.

Be assured that if your child is in a safe car seat, the chances of his getting injured in an accident are low.

Managing Medical Crises at Home

Staying calm while talking about what to do in an accident is much easier than staying calm if your child actually gets hurt. In this section we give you hints on how to stay calm and effective if your child needs help.

Don't panic! Don't panic!

Panic is inevitable when your child is injured, but try not to show it, because even babies can sense your alarm and respond to it with a few alarms of their own. Try to remember the following guidelines when your child crashes into the coffee table or experiences some other medical crisis:

✔ At first glance, it always looks like more blood than it actually is. Because blood is red, you notice it immediately. The injury probably isn't as bad as it first looks.

✔ Head and face wounds can bleed copiously because of the large number of blood vessels there. Clean up the area, and you may find just a tiny cut or scrape.

✔ Spurting blood can indicate a cut artery. Hold firm pressure over the wound with something clean. This injury requires medical attention, because arteries, unlike veins, don't stop spurting on their own quickly enough to prevent significant blood loss. Call 999.

✔ Any injury to the eye should be seen by an ophthalmologist. If your child has something stuck in his eye, don't pull it out; you may make things worse. Call 999.

✔ If you suspect a neck injury, don't move your child. Call 999 for help.

Calling the doctor

In an emergency, thinking clearly is very difficult. Sometimes you may even have trouble remembering your doctor's name, much less his phone number. To save yourself from fumbling through the phone book when you want to call your doctor, post the following information on your refrigerator in bold print so it's visible not only to you, but also to the babysitter, relative, friends or anyone else who may be watching the baby:

✔ **Your doctor's name and phone number:** Even you probably won't remember this information in an emergency.

✔ **Your baby's full name and date of birth:** Yes, we're sure you'll remember your baby's name. But today, with hyphenated last names and mums who keep their maiden names, don't be so sure your babysitter knows your baby's last name! And it's a pretty safe bet she doesn't know his date of birth, unless she's closely related to you.

✔ **Your address:** Believe it or not, people tend to go blank on this kind of information in an emergency. You may not forget where you live, but your mother-in-law may.

✔ **Your phone number:** Ditto the above. If she's got you on speed dial, your mother may not even know your phone number!

Taking the precaution of writing down important information may seem a little silly until you're actually in an emergency and can't seem to remember your own name, much less the baby's birth date.

When you get the doctor or accident and emergency personnel on the phone, speak clearly and slowly enough so they can understand you the first time and not waste time asking you to repeat yourself.

If you have the presence of mind to do so, jot down a few notes about exactly what happened, because, believe it or not, the actual details get very jumbled in a crisis, which is why eyewitness stories rarely match up.

Open Wide, Baby! Administering Medicine

Getting a baby to take medicine isn't as easy as it seems. Even small babies seem to have an uncanny sense that you've spiked their evening bottle with medicine.

When drawing up a dose of medication, remember that a kitchen teaspoon is not always a teaspoon; it can range from half a teaspoon to two or more. One teaspoon equals 5 millilitres or cubic centimetres, usually abbreviated to cc. Millilitres, known as ml, and cc are the same thing. So if the dose for your child's age is half a teaspoon, it's 2.5 ml or cc. To measure these minuscule amounts, you need a specially marked syringe, which pharmacies often routinely provide with medication. If yours doesn't, ask for one.

Since a wrestling match will end up with far more medication on your shirt and on the floor than in the baby, try the following tips when you really need your baby to take medicine:

- ✔ **Mix the medicine with a small amount of a sweet-tasting food like baby applesauce.** Unfortunately, even small amounts of medications often change the flavour of the food, so don't put a tiny bit of medicine into a large amount of food hoping to dilute the taste enough so that baby will eat it. He probably won't eat all the food, and you won't know how much medicine he actually got. Mix the medication into just a few bits of food the baby likes, and you may have a fighting chance of getting it into him.

- ✔ **If you mix medication into formula, don't spike the whole bottle, because this will be the first time in your baby's life that he doesn't chug down an entire 6 ounces of formula.** Mix it into 1 ounce, so he finishes it before he realises there's something odd going on.

- ✔ **Use a syringe to squirt the medicine into the baby's mouth.** Insert the syringe gently into the corner of his mouth; don't try to force his mouth wide open, unless you want to wear cherry-flavoured medicine for the rest of the day. Push the syringe plunger down slowly but steadily, gently holding his lips closed, and hope for the best.

- ✔ **Some medications can be given in rectal suppositories.** This may not sound like a really great solution, but inserting a suppository into the rectum is easier sometimes than getting medicine into a recalcitrant mouth. Just don't put a suppository into the child's mouth.

- ✔ **If your child is not an infant, firmly tell him he has to take his medicine.** You may not believe this now, but kids often know when you really mean business, and they comply. Obviously it's a miracle when it happens.

Taking a Baby's Temperature

Taking a baby's temperature is much easier now than it was a few years ago. You no longer have to stick a rigid glass thermometer into a flailing child's mouth and hold it there for three minutes – in fact, there are very good reasons not to! You can measure temperatures even in tiny babies much more easily today.

Choosing a thermometer

When standing in the big baby shop looking for items to add to your list, the sheer number of thermometer types may stagger you. Talking to friends who have babies may not clarify the thermometer choices either, because everyone seems to have a favourite method and hardly anyone agrees with anyone else. The following is a list of different types of thermometers and their pros and cons:

- **Digital rectal thermometers:** These are the gold standard for temperature taking, especially for infants younger than 3 months. Rectal thermometers measure internal temperature, the most accurate way to determine a child's temperature, and they have a flexible tip that gives if your child squirms. They're accurate and easy to use on some babies, although others hate them.

- **Digital oral thermometers:** These aren't practical or accurate until your child is 3 or 4 years old, because they can't hold them properly under their tongue and may bite and break them.

- **Axillary (under the arm) thermometer:** You can use a digital rectal or oral thermometer as an axillary thermometer, but this method gives the least accurate reading and normally registers as much as 2 degrees lower than a rectal temperature.

- **Tympanic thermometers:** These thermometers, shown in Figure 13-1, are used in the ear canal and aren't appropriate for use in children younger than 3 months because their ear canals are too small to properly insert the cone-shaped tip. They also may not be accurate for temperatures higher than 102°F (38.8°C).

- **Forehead thermometers:** These register temperature as you roll the tip across the forehead, but they're not very precise.

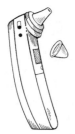

Figure 13-1: A tympanic ear thermometer.

Recognising fevers

So when is a fever a fever? It can be hard to know, especially when you're juggling half a dozen methods of temperature taking in an attempt to get an accurate reading. The following guidelines explain what your doctor means when he talks about a fever:

- ✔ **In an infant up to age 3 months, a rectal temperature of 100.4 °F (38 °C) or higher needs immediate evaluation.** Small babies don't normally run fevers, so even these seemingly low temperatures need attention.

- ✔ **Between ages 3 months and 3 years, a rectal fever of** 102 °F (38.8 °C) **or higher should be reported to your doctor.** Although fever is important, the way your child is behaving is equally significant. A child who is still eating, drinking and playing happily with a high fever is less concerning than a lethargic child with a lower fever.

- ✔ **Ear temperatures are roughly equivalent to rectal temperatures.** If you're sure the tip is properly inserted into the ear, call your doctor for a temperature of 100.4 °F (38 °C) for infants and 102 °F (38.8 °C) for ages 3 months to 3 years.

Febrile convulsions

Febrile convulsions are extremely scary for parents, although the child probably won't remember having one. Most febrile convulsions occur when the temperature rises suddenly, but the exact degree of fever isn't the determining factor of whether a child has one. Around 3 to 5 per cent of children experience febrile convulsions, usually between the ages of 5 months and 5 years.

Don't try to do anything while your child is having a convulsion, other than trying to cool him off by sponging him down with cool water. Don't put anything into his mouth or try to restrain him; more damage is done by these attempts to prevent damage.

Move any hard or sharp objects away from the child during a convulsion to prevent injury. Remember to move the objects away from the child; don't try to move the child away from the objects.

 Most febrile convulsions last only a few minutes, but your child may be limp and lethargic afterward. Follow up with your doctor immediately after a convulsion; he may want you to bring the baby in immediately or may be okay with a visit the next day to determine the cause of the high temperature. Be guided by his advice. Most parents who have just experienced an infant convulsion want the reassurance of a visit.

If your child's convulsion lasts 15 minutes or more, he starts to turn blue or he remains unresponsive after a convulsion, call 999 immediately.

Treating a fever

Fevers of 100.2 °F (37.8 °C) or less don't always need treatment. Fever is the body's way of fighting off infection, so giving your child medication at the first sign of a high temperature doesn't help his immune system to develop. Aspirin is no longer recommended for children because of the possibility of developing Reye's syndrome. Infants can be given children's paracetamol or ibuprofen in recommended doses.

Deciphering Nappy Contents

Some parents are inordinately interested in their offspring's waste products (mostly parents who were brought up to be inordinately obsessed with their own). But even parents who are pretty casual about the contents of a nappy can sometimes be concerned about what appears there.

Knowing what's normal

Breastfed babies normally have frequent stools that are often looser than those of bottle-fed babies. Breastfed babies' stools are often yellow and seedy, whereas bottle-fed babies' stools may be light brown and firmer.

Babies frequently poo after every feed in the first month or so, and then slow down production. Some babies may only 'produce' every few days, which is fine as long as the stool is soft. At the same time, they may begin to squirm, cry, grunt and make faces when pooing, worrying parents that they're having a hard time passing stools. What they're actually doing is becoming aware of their own bodily sensations.

However, if the stool is hard, comes out in pellets or if the baby doesn't go for several days, call your doctor for advice.

Checking out colour changes

Stools are usually yellowish or light brown respectively in babies who are exclusively breastfed and/or formula-fed. When unusual-coloured poo makes an appearance, parents are understandably concerned. Changes in stool colour can be perfectly normal or a sign of a problem, so keep the following information in mind when deciding whether to call the doctor:

- If your baby is on iron-fortified formula, he may have green or dark stools.

- Green stools can indicate an imbalance of foremilk, the first milk released, and hindmilk, which has a higher fat content. Too much foremilk and not enough hindmilk can produce green stools and upset the stomach. Allowing the baby to breastfeed long enough on one side – ten minutes or longer – to get a good dose of hindmilk corrects the problem.

- If blood is on the outside of the stool, the baby may have a small fissure and may need a stool softener, but ask the doctor. (Make sure the baby doesn't have a nappy rash that's causing the blood.)

- Bloody, mucousy stools need immediate attention, as they can indicate intestinal problems.

- Dark, tarry stools can indicate intestinal bleeding and should be evaluated.

Teething Symptoms and Remedies

Parents peer into their babies' mouths looking for teeth like gold miners sifting through the silt for nuggets of gold. When it comes to teeth, relaxing is the best thing you can do. All children, with very few exceptions, get teeth eventually, and prying your kid's mouth open to search for a pearly white doesn't make them come in any faster.

Keeping in mind that these guidelines have many exceptions, you generally can expect teeth to appear in this order and at these times:

- The first tooth appears between 4 and 7 months.

- The two lower middle teeth usually come in first.

- The two upper middle teeth follow next.

- The back teeth are the last to come, usually around age 2; you probably won't be all that excited by new teeth by then and may not even notice.

- By age 3, your child will have 20 teeth, 10 on each level.

After you get over the thrill of finding a new tooth, you may be consumed with ways to ease the discomfort of teething. Although alcohol, an old-fashioned remedy for easing the pain of teething, should not be applied to baby's gums, it may help to apply it to *yours*. You can decrease teething discomfort in your baby with:

- ✔ Pain medication such as paracetamol or ibuprofen.
- ✔ Teething gels applied to the gums.
- ✔ Chilled teething rings or other items for baby to bite down on.

Teething doesn't normally cause a temperature higher than 100°F (37.8 °C), so a fever still needs investigation, even if your baby is breaking in a full set of choppers all at once. (Not likely, by the way – teeth tend to trickle in no more than two at a time.) Teething can cause:

- ✔ Drooling.
- ✔ Irritability.
- ✔ Swollen gums.
- ✔ Difficulty sleeping.
- ✔ Difficulty nursing or taking a bottle.
- ✔ Biting on everything within reach.

Whether or not teething causes diarrhoea, vomiting and rashes other than the rashes associated with constant drooling is debatable. Children can get ill while teething, so don't assume that teething is responsible for sudden signs of illness.

Reacting to Medicines and Vaccines

Giving a child any type of foreign substance can trigger an allergic or hypersensitive reaction. New foods are actually the biggest culprit, but medications and vaccinations can also cause reactions.

Vaccination reactions – yours and your baby's

Many parents have concerns about the number of vaccinations given to infants and worry about which ones their child should have, when to give them and possible consequences of vaccinations. Remember that vaccines are given to prevent *serious* illness;

they're not given to prevent diseases that aren't potentially harmful for your child.

Giving two or three injections at one visit, especially when each one contains more than one vaccine, is concerning to many parents. But children are exposed to 2,000 to 6,000 antigens every day, as opposed to the 150 antigens introduced in vaccines during the entire vaccination schedule.

While no proof exists that vaccines are responsible for the increase in autism and similar issues, vaccines can cause complications in some children. Typical symptoms include a high temperature, pain at the injection site, redness or a rash. Approximately 3 out of 10,000 children have febrile convulsions (see the 'Recognising fevers' section earlier in this chapter for more on these) after getting the measles-mumps-rubella (MMR) vaccine.

The debate about how to spread out vaccines and which ones are really necessary could fill books – and undoubtedly has – and every couple has their own feelings about vaccines. The most important thing in deciding on how, when and what to vaccinate is to discuss the pros and cons with your doctor, and follow his recommendations.

Some children develop a rash after vaccinations. Again, if it lasts more than a day, ask the doctor about it.

Medications that cause reactions

Any medication can cause allergic reactions, but antibiotics are more likely to cause an adverse reaction. Typical offenders include:

- ✔ Penicillin or any of the same family, such as amoxicillin or ampicillin (penicillin causes more allergic reactions than any other antibiotic).
- ✔ Sulfa medications.
- ✔ Cephalosporins.

Drug allergies can cause a variety of skin reactions, including

- ✔ Rashes.
- ✔ Hives – small welts that move around from one area to another.
- ✔ Erythema multiforme, a moving bull's eye-patterned rash with a temperature, joint pains, itching and an overall sick feeling, as well as painful eyes and sore mouth.

Notify your doctor if any reaction occurs after taking any medication. Children's-strength chlorphenamine helps control itching and swelling in most cases, but follow your doctor's advice. Severe reactions may require steroids.

Dealing with Food Allergies

Food allergies affect around 1 in 18 babies before the age of 3. As with many facets of baby-raising, the thinking on solid food introduction and allergies has completely changed since you were a baby, a fact that can result in heated discussions between you and your parents.

Introducing new foods

At one time, introducing solids early was all the rage in parenting, as if having your 2-month-old chow down pureed carrots merited some sort of parenting prize. Today, paediatricians recommend waiting until a baby is around 6 months old to introduce new foods to reduce the chance of developing food allergies, especially the five most common food allergens, which are:

- Cow's milk.
- Eggs.
- Peanuts.
- Soya.
- Wheat.

An almost unbelievable 90 per cent of food allergies are caused by one of these big five. The age at which the food is first introduced is no longer considered a factor in whether a child develops allergies after the age of six months.

Recognising allergic reactions

Parents who have allergies themselves may be looking for signs of allergies in their children, and allergic tendencies do run in families. Some common reactions are in fact intolerances not allergies, like reddened cheeks after eating tomatoes or citrus fruits. Lactose intolerance, caused by a missing enzyme that breaks down milk products, also isn't an allergy. Irritability, skin rashes and intestinal upsets are the most common signs of food allergy in infants (and signs of food intolerances as well, which they can grow out of).

Colic, skin rashes and stomach upsets such as loose stools are the most common signs of food allergy or intolerance, but severe anaphylactic reactions with difficulty breathing, hives and loss of consciousness can also occur, often within minutes of eating the offending food. Get medical help immediately if this occurs.

Having previously eaten a food without a reaction is no guarantee that an allergic reaction won't occur; reactions don't always occur the first time a person is exposed to a substance. Always call your doctor if a significant reaction occurs and follow his recommendations on treatment.

Preventing allergic reactions

The best prevention for allergy development is exclusive breast-feeding for at least the first 4 to 6 months of life. Some evidence exists for prevention of wheezing in infancy and early childhood by exclusive breastfeeding for the first 3 months of life. There's no proof that use of soya formulas prevents allergies compared to cow's milk-based formulas; in fact, many children with cow's milk allergies are also allergic to soya.

Cook fruits and vegetables for your baby rather than serving them raw, because cooking appears to decrease the risk of allergic reactions. Processed foods, including junior baby foods, contain a number of ingredients, which makes it hard to tell what an infant is reacting to if he develops an allergic reaction.

If your child has severe allergies, your doctor may recommend carrying an Epi-pen injector containing adrenaline in case of serious allergic reaction. Fortunately, around 20 per cent of children outgrow allergies and intolerance to foods by the time they hit school age.

Chapter 14

Time and Money: The High Cost of Having a Baby

*E*ven before baby arrived you probably never felt like you had enough time in the day or money in the bank for everything you wanted to do. Money concerns aren't a new worry in the lives of most new parents, but with nappies, baby wipes and the cutest clothing you've ever seen in your life added to your weekly expenses, even financially sound parents can quickly begin to feel strapped for cash.

The only thing in shorter supply than money may be your time. Sometimes just finding the time to shower in the morning may feel like a major accomplishment, but keeping your life and self in order is important for your entire family. Adjusting to a new life in which baby comes first is a challenge, and even the most organised parents will find that tasks that used to require minimal effort are now a major undertaking. In this chapter we take a look at how to juggle your new responsibilities with your old ones – with a little fun mixed in to boot.

Creating a New Work/Life Balance with Baby

Unfortunately, bliss doesn't pay the bills, which means that unless you're embarking on a new journey as a stay-at-home dad or you win the lottery while on paternity leave, you'll find yourself back in the throes of work in what feels like the blink of an eye. Don't be surprised if for the first few days you find yourself disinterested, distracted or bored on the job, especially if your partner is still at home. In the beginning your mind will be more focused on the amazing event you've just experienced, and the fatigue your brain may be feeling as a result of less sleep won't help any.

When you're working full time again, winding down after a hard day won't be as easy as it once was now that you have to help with baby's bath-time, night feeds, nappy changes and endless chores. Congratulations – you now have another full-time job awaiting you when you get home.

Striking an ideal work/life balance is a major challenge for all parents, and it takes a lot of negotiating, planning and sacrifice. From work to home to play, everything becomes a little more complicated to juggle. In the following sections we help you make the best of a very full plate.

Taking time off with paternity leave

Not so very long ago, new dads were expected back on the job the day after welcoming a baby into the world. And although we're still a long way from equal time off for both mother and father, strides have been made to allow new dads time to bond with their new family.

To qualify for Ordinary Paternity Leave, you must tell your employer when the baby is due (or when the child is expected to be placed with you for adoption), whether you want one or two weeks' leave and when you want this leave to start.

You also need to give your employer the correct amount of notice. You should tell them in writing at least 15 weeks before the beginning of the week when the baby is due.

One of the simplest ways to give paternity notice is to fill in a 'self-certificate'. You can download form SC3, 'Becoming a Parent', from www.direct.gov.uk.

Your Ordinary Paternity Leave can start on any day of the week (but not before the baby is born) and has to finish within 56 days of the baby's birth. If the baby is born before the week she is due, Ordinary Paternity Leave must finish within 56 days of the first day of that week. You can start Ordinary Paternity Leave after a period of parental leave has ended.

If your partner has a multiple birth, you are still only allowed one period of Ordinary Paternity Leave.

Additional paternity leave (APL) is a recent development, which allows an employee to take up to 26 weeks' leave on top of the two weeks of Ordinary Paternity Leave. This can only be taken 20 weeks or more after the child's birth, and once the mother has returned to work from statutory maternity leave or ended her entitlement. To qualify for APL, a father must have been on a continuous contract with his employer for at least 26 weeks by the end of the 15th week before the baby is due.

Discussing your leave options

Before meeting with your employers to find out what arrangements for leave you can make, speak with other recent fathers in your company about their experiences to get a better idea of what to expect. Their information can provide you with an opportunity to craft a plan that meets your needs and adheres to your company's policies. Some great questions to ask other fathers are:

- ✔ What was the company's paternity leave policy at the time you became a new dad?

- ✔ How did your boss react to your paternity leave inquiry?

- ✔ How much time off was granted? How much of it was paid?

- ✔ How did you structure your paternity leave?

- ✔ Did you ask about using flexitime before or after baby's arrival? If so, what was the response?

- ✔ How much responsibility did you have to take for covering your job in your absence?

- ✔ What is the one thing you wish you had done differently in arranging your time off?

When meeting with your boss and/or HR representative, make sure to take notes of everything that is said and get any policy-related statements in writing. In addition to asking about some of the issues in the questions above, be sure to ask about the company's policy regarding additional time off in case of complications with mum or baby.

Getting all your paperwork in order

Be sure to get the necessary time-off paperwork in order prior to heading to the hospital. Don't get defensive if your employer requires a doctor's note regarding your leave – nobody is questioning the fact that you're a new parent, but rules must be followed.

Managing sick leave when you're back at work

When both parents head back to work, sick leave suddenly becomes a hot commodity. Between baby's multitude of doctor appointments, vaccination reactions, high temperatures and diarrhoea, as well as your babysitter's unexpected crises, you may be required to leave work more frequently than you used to do pre-baby.

Check with your employer several weeks prior to the beginning of your leave to find out if flexitime or working-at-home days are allowed in case of child illness or childcare gaps. If they aren't, remain honest. Don't start coughing and sneezing or fabricate some family emergency as a front to mask the real reason you have to leave.

Ask for a performance evaluation a month or so after returning from paternity leave. If you're experiencing bouts of insecurity and anxiety about how you're perceived and performing on the job now that you're a dad, or feel intimated or scared about asking for days off because of the new baby, a performance review gives you an opportunity to address any minor issues that have arisen before they become fully-fledged annoyances for your boss. Be sure to let your boss know that you're aware that your schedule is trickier than normal, and that you appreciate some flexibility as you adjust to the new situation. Letting your boss know that you're open to criticism and want to fix any problems will make you look like the responsible new parent you've become.

Dealing with after-work expectations

Depending on the business you're in, you may be used to participating in after-work activities and commitments. However, after baby arrives, it quickly becomes clear that you no longer have the ability to attend happy hour three nights a week. Although nobody wants to be seen as the new dad who suddenly says no to everything and isn't the same fun, karaoke-loving guy he used to be, a certain amount of reality will dictate your ability to party instead of heading straight home to spend time with your family.

Evaluate any after-work requests using the following guidelines to help you determine the appropriate way to handle them:

✔ **Mandatory engagements:** Sometimes meetings run late, business dinners take priority and your boss asks you to work overtime on a very important project. Always say yes to anything that's important to the function and maintenance of your job, and work with your partner to find help for her at home if needed.

✔ **Occasionally important dates:** A beer isn't always just a beer. Sometimes going to a pub after work is an important networking opportunity or even where important business decisions are made and advancement opportunities created. Try not to commit to quasi-important after-work requests more than a few times each month.

✔ **Optional events:** Sometimes a beer *is* just a beer – and there's nothing wrong with that, as long as you keep in mind that you can say yes only so many times without annoying your partner and it's best to save those for when it really counts. If you perceive an after-work event to be merely for sport, pass unless you need a mental-health night out. Just remember that every time you say yes, you're giving your partner the opportunity to say yes to an activity of her own down the road. It doesn't take too many commitments to severely diminish that all-important family time.

Be proactive in scheduling out-of-the-office social events over lunch. If you take the lead, you'll have control over when they're held and won't feel the need to justify your inability to commit to activities after work.

If colleagues challenge your decision to not attend after-work events that you perceive to be nothing more than social calls, don't feel the need to defend your decision. Let them know that you spend eight hours a day with your colleagues and you like to spend the rest with your family.

Reprioritising your commitments

With so much on your plate, you may wonder when you'll have time to hit the gym, go to the cinema, take your partner on a date, volunteer at the local farmers' market or engage in any of the myriad activities you enjoy doing. The bad news is that there isn't time in the day/week/month to do everything you've always done on top of caring for baby. The good news is that you'll still have time to have fun despite your over-full schedule.

Make sure to keep yourself high on the list of priorities, because you can't manage work, family and your social life if you're run down, ill or depressed. If you try to do it all, you won't do anything very well because you'll be spread too thin. To have more energy and stave off illness, take your vitamins, get as much sleep as possible, eat healthy foods and continue to make exercise a priority.

Just as you wouldn't skip a doctor's appointment or just not show up at work one day, you have to schedule your personal commitments as well. Whether that's a stroll through the park with your family, sex with your partner or time to sit and watch a tennis match on TV, don't make your personal time optional or the balance between work and life can easily become off kilter.

How do you make the work/life balance stay in balance? Keep a calendar and write down everything, even blocking out time you set aside for fun. Try as best as you can to separate your commitments by focusing on work at work, family during family time and you during your scheduled personal time. You can't make the most of your time if you're mentally juggling too many tasks and people.

Figuring out what's most important to you

Because thinking about everything you need and want to do at the same time is impossible, make a list of all your commitments and activities. Your list may include the following activities:

- ✔ Spending time with your family
- ✔ Working overtime
- ✔ Exercising
- ✔ Socialising with friends
- ✔ Engaging in hobbies
- ✔ Travelling
- ✔ Maintaining a healthy relationship with your partner
- ✔ Helping with community clubs
- ✔ Participating in clubs and team sports

When you complete your list, ask yourself, 'If I could only give my attention to one thing in life, what would that be?' After you pick the most important thing in your life, choose the next four so you've designated your top five priorities. As your child grows and your life changes, frequently revisit this priority list. What's important to you now may not be as important four months from now.

Figuring out what can go, at least for now

After you set your priorities, drop any unnecessary activities from your to-do list – at least the ones that require a major time commitment. Sure, a twice-weekly 5-a-side league may be fun but is it really vital to your well-being and that of your family? How much TV can you cut out of your week and still feel entertained? Any activity that eats up copious amounts of your time without much reward should be removed from your regular routine.

Work with your partner, as well as babysitters and family members, to help you adhere to your priority list. Couples often relay to great effect: mum watches baby while dad attends guitar lessons, and dad watches baby while mum goes to yoga. And when your friends and family members offer to babysit, try not to always use that time for errands. Instead, take your partner out for a night – or an afternoon, which is sometimes easier with babies – on the town.

Readjusting When and If Mum Goes Back to Work

Not every mother (or father, for that matter!) decides to go back to work. Some have to do so for financial reasons even when their hearts and tear ducts tell them otherwise. And some mothers and fathers are excited to get back to the daily routine and job they love. Everyone's experience is different, but regardless of what choice you and your partner make, the transition is challenging.

Making going back to work easier on mum

Mum gets far more time off work after baby is born than you will, which only makes the going-back process more difficult and emotional for her. There may be tears, running mascara, threats of quitting her job – lots of them – and it's your job to support her through this difficult transition.

Mum's innate protective instincts will be at an all-time high the moment she's forced to put her 3-month-old baby into a nursery or with a childminder for 40-plus hours every week. When you went back to work, you had the benefit of making the transition when baby was at home with the only other person you trust as much as yourself to care for her. Under most circumstances, mum doesn't get that luxury, and taking the leap back into business-as-usual won't be easy for her.

Try these techniques to ease your partner's return to the workplace:

✔ **Practise in advance:** Getting out the door won't ever be the same again, and the last thing you want is a panicked, rushed mum on her first day back. Much like you did with the trial run to the hospital before baby's birth, take the time to go through a trial run for mum's first day back to work. It will benefit you, too, since you'll be involved in the process of getting baby fed and clothed and delivered to the nursery or childminder *and* still making it to work on time.

✔ **Provide mummy alone time:** It's not so unusual for new mums to cling to their newborns, and in some cases, going back to work is your partner's first separation experience after giving birth. Start slowly by giving your partner blocks of time to be alone at the weekend or in the evening during which she can practise doing things without baby around.

✔ **Get comfortable with childcare:** Trusting someone else to care for your fragile baby isn't easy, but the sooner you start, the easier it will be when that care becomes more frequent. Start letting friends and family take short shifts watching the baby, and even ask your future childcare provider to take on a shift before your partner goes back to work. Also, feel free to ask your provider for time to observe her interaction with your child, be that at the nursery or childminder's home.

✔ **Stagger the return:** Going from full-time mum to full-time employee overnight can be a major shock to the system. Get your partner to talk to her employer about the possibility of a staggered return. If the first week back she only works one day, and then the following week she works three, and so on, the transition will be much smoother.

✔ **Plan ahead for morning:** Mornings are tough for everyone, so don't leave anything other than showering and getting dressed for first thing because you now have to factor in getting baby ready for the day and travel time to the nursery or childminder's home. Take time the night before to make lunches, pick out clothing, pack baby's nappy bag and so on to create a calmer mood in the morning.

If your partner is threatening to quit her job the first day back, don't panic and certainly don't try to change her mind. The best thing to do is listen to her concerns and give her all the bonding time she needs with baby upon returning home from work. Tell her to take it day by day, and that at the end of every week you'll re-evaluate the situation. There's nothing wrong with her making the decision to stay at home, but making the decision when her emotions are heightened isn't a good idea.

Following are some thoughtful ways to improve your partner's emotional state during the transition back to work:

- ✔ **Digitise baby:** Buy your partner a digital picture frame for her desk at work, or even a pocket-sized device if she works in a non-office environment. Add new pictures every day to give your partner a daily visual fix of baby.

- ✔ **Free nights for bonding:** Though you won't want to shoulder the chore burden all by yourself forever, consider giving your wife a get-out-of-jail-free card during her first week back. Allow her to spend every waking moment with baby to give her the opportunity to reconnect with her child and not feel like she's missing out on everything.

- ✔ **Shower her with gifts and praise:** You don't have to go overboard, but some flowers on her first day back may go a long way toward making her smile, at least for a second, during that first week back. Be sure to tell her how well she's doing at adjusting to the changes and that you think she's a wonderful mother.

- ✔ **Don't try to fix it:** Let her cry and validate her experience, even if you don't understand why it's so hard. Mothers give birth to the babies, and as deep as the bond between fathers and kids can run, it's still different for mum. Call her throughout the day to check in and let her know that what she's experiencing is normal.

Deciding to be a stay-at-home parent

Making the decision to be a stay-at-home parent can be the fulfilment of a lifelong dream for some parents and a total surprise to others. If you and your partner make the decision that one of you will stay at home to care for baby, thus begins another exciting, challenging chapter in your new parenthood experience. However, it isn't a decision that should be taken lightly. If you've been used to receiving income from both yourself and your partner, losing half that income will make a profound difference to your lives, and you and your partner need to consider carefully whether or not you can make it work.

Considering whether your partner can stay at home

Some women know in advance that they don't want to go back to work after having a baby, and some come to that decision after baby arrives. If you can make it work financially and your partner is refusing to budge, do your best to make arrangements for her to stay at home that work for both of you. She may have loved her job before and you thought the routine you'd established as a family was working fine, but while you don't always need to understand why your partner feels the way she does, it's vital that you respect her right to feel that way. Take plenty of time to talk it over and make sure staying home is really a feasible option.

Looking at options when you can't afford to lose the income

Sometimes the desire to stay at home won't subside, and you and your partner may be at odds as to what's best for your family. If your financial situation doesn't allow for your household income to be reduced by thousands of pounds annually, stand your ground. Be understanding of her concerns and desires, but don't risk your financial security in order to make her happy. Most importantly, don't rule it out forever. Make a savings plan that you both can work toward in order to achieve her goal of staying at home. Encourage your partner to seek out working-at-home opportunities. Work with your partner to create a tangible goal that will keep your finances in the black and eventually allow her to stay at home.

Sometimes both parents want to quit their jobs to stay at home and care for the child. Unless you and your partner are independently wealthy, this won't be an option. As unfortunate as it is, the decision will probably come down to money. If you can only afford for one person to stay at home, the logical choice is for the person with the larger salary to continue working. It's possible, however, that the person who makes more money is working long hours and travelling frequently. Sometimes the decision is better made from a work/life balance standpoint rather than salary. In this case, lifestyle changes have to make up for the loss of salary – but it can be done.

Some companies are adapting to the push for flexibility by allowing new parents the opportunity to spend some or all of their working hours at home. This arrangement can ease your partner's pain if she really wants to stay at home with baby but you can't afford to lose her income. However, working at home doesn't eliminate the need for childcare; you still need someone in the home to help while your partner gets work done, unless your partner is willing to work nights and weekends while you take over childcare duties. Even then, having babysitters at the ready is a must for busy times, meetings and phone conferences.

If you and your partner can both work from home, you may be able to stagger your working hours so that you take turns caring for the baby. These kinds of alternate work arrangements can vary widely; your company may have guidelines in place for such arrangements, or you may have to create your own plan and then negotiate for its acceptance. Ask your boss or human resources manager about this option if you're interested.

Helping mum adjust if she doesn't go back to work

The adjustment to being a stay-at-home mum can be just as challenging as heading back to work, only in different ways. As wonderful as it is to have the opportunity to raise your own child during the day, it can be an isolating experience. Some women will find themselves a bit stir-crazy from all of the indoor time and begin to crave adult interaction.

Here are some ways to help your partner transition to staying at home:

- ✔ **Repeat after us: bringing up a child is a job.** Sure, staying at home may seem at times like a dream job – access to the TV all day, no more commuting – but resist the thought that she's got it made. As you know full well by now, taking care of a baby is exhausting. Babies require full-time attention and are the most demanding bosses on earth.

- ✔ **Remember that her office is your home.** If your partner suddenly has higher standards for the cleanliness and tidiness of your home, help her keep it that way. She's now in the house all day, every day, and as strange as it may sound, you need to treat your home as her office, too.

- ✔ **Encourage hobbies.** Mental boredom is inevitable, no matter how much your partner loves your child. Stacking Lego, reading books and taking long walks can be fun, but urge your partner to take up a hobby that's just for her that works her mind and gives her something to focus on other than baby.

- ✔ **Give her personal time.** When you get home from work, you'll both need some time to unwind from a long day. Make sure to give her as much time off from baby duty as she needs. Plan relaxing surprises for her, such as a massage, every once in a while to make sure her emotional needs are being met. Work together to create an evening schedule that allows both of you ample baby-free time. Alternate being responsible for bath-time, reading, the bedtime routine and so on, to give both of you free time to relax. Just because you're away from baby all day doesn't mean that you should be the sole caregiver once you get home.

✔ **Ask her about her day.** Just because she's not in meetings and dealing with bosses doesn't mean she won't need to talk about the challenges and events of the day. Be sure to ask how she's doing – it's easy to do, but easy to forget.

✔ **Don't think of her as your maid/errand girl.** Just because she's home all day doesn't mean picking up your dry cleaning, making dinner, food shopping and hoovering are all her responsibilities. She has more time to do things around the house, but don't give her a list of things to do for you. Being a stay-at-home mum doesn't mean you're her boss. Thank her profusely for everything she does that benefits both of you every day.

Some days you hate your job, and the same rings true for the stay-at-home parent. Imagine how you'd feel if you never got a day off from your job. A stay-at-home parent works every day and nights and weekends too, so if your partner reaches boiling point, don't hesitate to offer her a day off. Either take a day's leave to stay home or encourage your partner to find alternate childcare for the day.

You may be surprised how much stress will be removed from your life when your partner transitions to full-time childcare and can do some of the chores and tasks that eat up your precious weekend, but don't have unrealistic expectations. Taking care of a baby is a full-time job as it is. To help both of you adjust to her stay-at-home schedule, sit down together and work out what her new role will look like so that you expect the same things. Create a 'job description' that will benefit the entire family and help avoid frustration down the road, and be open to modifying it if she discovers that, say, doing all the laundry and cooking in addition to her childcare duties is exhausting her.

Becoming a stay-at-home dad

By no means is the stay-at-home dad a norm yet. If you decide to stay at home, remember that the rules outlined for the stay-at-home mum are no different to the rules for you.

Following are some special considerations for the stay-at-home dad:

✔ **Fight for your right to 'daddy'.** If you've never experienced sexism, get ready for an onslaught. As a stay-at-home dad, at every turn you'll be confronted by people who are surprised at your choice, concerned that you don't know what you're doing and judgemental regarding your decision to 'throw away' your career. Strangers, especially women, will fawn over you and even say that it's so nice of you to 'babysit' for mum. Be confident in your decision and let the world know that you're excited about your new career and that men are capable of more than changing a nappy. Taking care of a baby is a lot of hard work, but it's not rocket science – you can do it!

✔ **Make friends with other parents.** Be it mums at the park or daddy playgroups, reach out to other stay-at-home parents in your neighbourhood even before the baby comes. You'll need friends to lean on for advice and last-minute babysitting, and the more you help out your new-parent friends and neighbours, the more options for help you'll have when you need it.

✔ **Utilise your unique skills.** Babies are mesmerised by everything, so use your stay-at-home time as an opportunity to play guitar, further your baking skills or even start a home-based business. Having a daytime activity will provide you with a much-needed creative outlet and, down the road, your kid will learn to appreciate (and mimic) your skills.

✔ **Turn off the TV.** It's tempting to keep the box on in the background all day, but too much TV isn't good for babies and children. Limit your TV time to two hours or less a day while baby is awake. Naptime is all yours.

Exploring the Expected (And Unexpected) Costs of Baby

One of the first things you'll hear from other parents is how expensive it is to have and bring up a child in today's high-cost world. Some costs of having a child are fixed and can't be avoided. Babies need food, clothes, nappies, wipes and a safe, warm place to sleep. Babies don't need an entire wardrobe jam-packed with enough designer-label clothing to make the Beckhams weep with envy. You and your partner need to control the urge to shower your baby with every possible toy or accessory.

The following sections help guide you in spending your money wisely on only the things baby truly must have.

Deciding what baby really needs

Experts estimate that baby's first year of life, including childcare, nappies and clothing, just to name a few, will cost you about £8,500 – and far more if you live in a city where childcare costs are usually greater. You'll quickly find that the choices you make with your cash have to count.

After you bring baby home, her needs are rather modest, but the costs will add up very quickly if you don't stick to the basics. Before you run out and buy the baby bouncy chair, swing, play mat and so on, spend some time getting to know what your baby likes so you won't be stuck with a lot of unused toys that cost you a lot of money.

 Most towns have a nearly new shop for baby equipment and car boot sales are a good source of baby clothing. One thing you'll quickly learn is that the lifespan of baby goods long outlasts the amount of time your child will actually use them, and there's nothing wrong with buying used items instead of new. Just make sure that what you buy is clean, in good condition and meets current safety standards. Some things, for example mattresses and car seats, you might not want to buy secondhand, unless you've checked the item out meticulously. Buying secondhand is a great way to get inexpensive clothing, toys and buggies, especially since your baby will grow out of all of them before you know it.

Network with the other parents you know, especially those with older babies or toddlers born in the same season as your baby. Many parents will happily pass along or sell you the things they no longer use, which simultaneously frees up space in their home and cuts down on the cost for you.

Whenever possible, before you buy anything, give your child the chance to try it out. Pull down the shop sample or take it out of the box to make sure your child is engaged with what you're about to buy. You may think all bouncy chairs are the same, but your baby inevitably will like one more than another. To make sure you get your money's worth, buy what your baby shows interest in.

Bracing yourself for the costs of must-have baby supplies

Babies don't need a lot of stuff, but what they do need tends to be a bit on the expensive side. If your partner isn't breastfeeding, you'll have to spend a great deal of money on formula, which is quite expensive. Parents opting to use only organic, chemical-free goods for their baby will find the costs increase as well.

Every choice you make will change the weekly amount you spend, but here's a basic look at what to expect:

✔ **Nappies and wipes:** If you develop an allegiance to a particular brand of disposable nappies, you're going to spend around £10 every week. Many supermarkets offer their own brands, which can cut the cost in half. Baby wipes present the same conundrum, with the name-brand options costing around £12 for a month's supply.

For both nappies and wipes, the cost-per-unit goes down when you buy a larger-sized box. You're going to be using wipes for the foreseeable future, but baby will outgrow nappies, so make sure not to buy a box that may go to waste. Also, buy only what you have room to store – it's worth a little extra to not have a house overfilled with nappies and wipes.

Upfront costs are higher for cloth nappies than disposable, but you'll save money in the long run. How much cheaper depends on the type you buy and how you wash them.

Your baby will be in nappies for around two and a half years, and using disposables for that time will cost approximately £600. Cloth nappies will cost around £250 to buy. Washing them over a two-and-a-half-year period will cost approximately £80. So the total cost of using cloth nappies is around £330, providing a saving of around £270. Bear in mind, however, that if you tumble dry your baby's nappies you could add over £100 to your bill. You can really save with cloth nappies if you plan to have more children. By using your nappies again, you dramatically reduce your overall costs.

✔ **Feeding supplies:** Whether your partner breastfeeds or uses formula, you'll have costs to meet.

• **Breastfeeding supplies:** Breast milk may be free, but you still need supplies, especially if mum is going back to work. Aside from a decent breast pump (a one-time cost of anything from £20 to over £200 depending on whether you want a simple manual pump or an all-singing, all-dancing electronic one), you'll also need freezer storage bags and breast pads (for leakages) for a while.

• **Formula:** Expect to spend around £7 for a 2-pound (900g) tin of powdered cow's milk-based formula, which lasts about a week. You generally pay about the same for soya-based infant formulas and lactose-free formulas. Hydrolysed-protein formula costs more, although you can get this on prescription if your baby is intolerant of or allergic to cow's milk. Speciality formulas, including those for sensitive systems and organic brands, cost even more.

✔ **Clothing and laundry:** Baby-safe washing powder costs more than the stuff you buy for your own clothes, and you'll have to use it for the first 18 to 24 months of baby's life. And, seeing as babies grow at a rapid pace, you need to allot around £25 to £75 per month to clothing, which includes hats, shoes, babygros, coats, socks and outfits so cute they could make a puppy bark with jealousy.

Some parents opt to use dye-free washing powder that's intended for adult use. Using these detergents for the whole family will simplify the laundry process and save you money. Make sure to read the label of any product to make sure it's non-toxic. Also, for babies with sensitive skin, use a dash of vinegar in the wash cycle in lieu of fabric softener.

You can save money on clothing by checking out charity shops and car boot sales and asking for hand-me-downs from friends with older children. All babies outgrow clothes before they're worn out, so you can find a lot of perfectly good used items at a fraction of the cost of new.

University may seem a long way off, but it's never too early to start saving for your child's education. However, if you don't have a retirement fund or an emergency fund for your own future survival, start there. You have to take care of your future first, and that responsibility sets a good example for your child. And if you can't pay for that university education someday, well, that's what student loans are for!

Comparing childcare options and costs

Paying someone else to care for your child for 40 hours each week will become your new number-one expense. In fact, depending on where you live, childcare may very well cost you more than your mortgage or rent. Taking care of a baby is big business, but it's also a huge responsibility, so it comes with an equally huge financial burden.

Just like shopping for cars, you have many options when choosing childcare. Depending on whether you're looking to buy a luxury car (a nanny) or a two-door runaround (the childminder up the road) or something in between, the costs will vary depending on the services you're promised.

Regardless of which option you choose, create a contract (unless the provider has one of her own) to make sure you're getting what you expect and that you won't have unexpected costs when you pay the bill. Go over the following questions with your childcare provider and get the answers in writing:

✔ Are you a registered childminder or is this nursery registered?

✔ What training have you received in childcare and education? What about your staff?

✔ Are you insured in case of accidents?

✔ Who is providing the food?

✔ How often and on what day are you expected to pay?

✔ Do you need my permission to take my child in a car?

✔ How much notice do you or I need to give in order to terminate the agreement?

✔ Do you frequently have visitors? Are they allowed to interact with the children?

✔ Will my child always be under your care, or will your spouse/child/friend/family member be helping?

✔ Do I have to pay when my child is unwell or we are on holiday?

✔ How do you discipline children?

✔ What do you charge for days when I need to drop my child off early/pick her up late?

✔ What security provisions are in place?

✔ Are you certified in both infant and child resuscitation?

✔ What is the carer to child ratio? (For childminders, ask how many other children are cared for and what their ages are.)

You should visit the nursery premises and get an idea of the types of facilities, toys and activities available.

Outlining your expectations in writing will reduce your fears and help prevent any unexpected surprises down the road.

If, after you check out the costs of childcare, you're reconsidering quitting your job (or having your partner quit her job) and staying at home, be sure to carefully weigh the points outlined in the 'Deciding to be a stay-at-home parent' section, earlier in this chapter. Staying at home is expensive in its own way and isn't a decision to be made lightly.

Childminder

A childminder is probably your cheapest option. Childminders must be registered with their local authority and have undergone a CRB (Criminal Records Bureau) check. They are also inspected by Ofsted on an annual basis.

Nursery

A nursery accommodates many children and employs multiple staff members to care for them. Nurseries are generally divided into small age-specific rooms, with individual staff assigned to each age group. The average yearly expenditure for 25 hours of nursery care per week for a child under two stands at £5,028 in England, £5,178 in Scotland and £4,723 in Wales.

Nanny

Paying someone to come into your home to provide full-time child-care for your child and your child alone is a very expensive option. For many parents, the peace of mind involved in this set-up is worth every penny, especially when you factor in the time, petrol and stress saved by not having to take your child to the nursery or childminder every day. Costs vary, depending on your location, the nanny's level of experience and the number of hours she's expected to be in your home.

Managing Your Money

Regardless of your financial situation, the impact of a baby will be felt early and often. Aside from the frightening amount of supplies, toys and clothing, the enormous cost of childcare will leave you with a lot less cash – and financial freedom – than you had in the past. Depending on where you live and the option you choose, you may be paying your childcare provider between £300 and £450 every week!

So perhaps your days of £3 skinny lattes are behind you. Maybe you'll be buying one less album online each month. Regardless of your vices and other financial obligations, you'll need to get your spending habits in tip-top shape to absorb the high cost of having children.

Prioritising your needs

The difference between what you want and what you need is a gulf roughly the size of the English Channel. The same can be said for what you want for your baby and what your baby actually needs in order to thrive. As a parent you have to get the needs of your entire family in check to secure a financially sound future for all.

Every family's situation and needs are different, but one rule is universal: make a budget. Start by taking a realistic look at where your money goes. Go through your bank account and credit card statements and work out how you spent your money in the past year. If you struggle to make cuts, consider meeting with a financial advisor. Figuring out how to spend, save and survive is a big job, and you don't have to go it alone.

Factor in the monthly costs of housing, food, transportation, investments, insurance and any medicines you take regularly. You also have to plan for the unexpected, and with a baby in the equation you'll have a lot of unexpected. Starting an emergency fund is easier said than done, but it's a must. When you have a kid, absorbing an unexpected job loss, income reduction or family emergency can be debilitating. Try to slowly work your way up to having six months' expenses set aside just in case life throws you a googly.

It is unpleasant to think about tragedy, but now is the time to make sure you have sufficient life insurance coverage for you, your partner and your baby. Work with a reputable insurance agent to make sure that your family will be provided for if the worst were to happen. Also, make sure that you have short- and long-term disability coverage through your employer. If not, consider buying your own policy. See Chapter 15 for more on insurance and disability coverage.

Determining where to cut costs

Giving up things you love isn't easy, but it's a must now that you have someone to provide for. Consider cutting costs in the following areas:

- ✔ **Food:** Pre-packaged and/or snack foods tend to be expensive. Items such as chips, ice cream, sweets, beer, frozen dinners and fizzy drinks are not only bad for your body, but also bad for your budget. You may not be willing to give them up all together, but try to cut down on the number of purchases of these high-cost, low-nutrition foods. Also, consider making a big casserole or stew to eat for numerous meals, which will reduce both your time in the kitchen and your food bill.

- ✔ **Utilities/bills:** Take a long, hard look at your monthly expenses. Do you need both a mobile and a home phone? Can you downgrade any of your contracts to a lower-cost option that still suits your needs? Can you go on a monthly payment plan to evenly spread out the costs of heating your home throughout the year? Are you in good standing with your credit card company? If so, ask to reduce your interest rate. Call every insurance company you do business with and see if you can get a lower rate. Don't be afraid to ask all of the companies that you do regular business with for a financial break.

✔ **Entertainment:** Take a look at the last six months of expenses and try to cut out or reduce the monthly cost of these non-essential items, which are the biggest expendable category for cost savings. Cable TV is not a utility, and if you're struggling to make ends meet, consider cutting your package down to basic or even getting rid of it altogether, even just for a little while. If you have both cable and a mail-based film subscription, do you truly need both? Baby will automatically limit the times you can go out to dinner, see a film or attend a football match, but monitor and limit these expenses, too, especially if you have to pay for a babysitter when you go out.

✔ **Convenience purchases:** Yes, buying lunch is simpler than getting up early to make it in the morning. Same goes for coffee. If you find yourself a constant consumer of takeout food, taxis, dry cleaning, bottled water and other non-essential costs that simply make your life easier, cut back. Even one less purchase per month can make a major impact on your bank account.

Turn to Chapter 15 to find out more about budgeting and cutting costs.

Chapter 15

Planning for Your New Family's Future

· ·

In This Chapter

▶ Organising your finances and putting safety nets in place

▶ Saving for your child's education

▶ Buying life insurance for worst-case scenarios

▶ Creating a will and designating a guardian for your child

· ·

During this time of immense joy, you probably resist worrying about the ifs, ands or buts that could bring all of that happiness to a screeching halt. You may also think it seems a bit premature to begin squirrelling away cash for his education when your baby hasn't even mastered the art of sitting up. But, as the time-honoured cliché goes, they grow up so fast.

Planning for the future, whether for planned events or unexpected ones, is the least enjoyable part of being a parent because it reminds you just how fleeting life can be. And nobody wants to think about what would happen if they died, especially with a newborn just beginning to enhance life. However, now is the time to make sure your child will be taken care of, regardless of the circumstances.

Securing a Financially Sound Future

New parents are saddled with an enormous increase in caretaking responsibilities. In fact, your role as caretaker now involves getting your financial life in order so that you can properly care for your child today, tomorrow and even after you and your partner die. It's not the cheeriest item on the new-parent to-do list, but it's one of the top priorities.

In this section we share some financial tips that will help to ensure a bright (and green!) future for your entire family.

Prioritise your expenses

Singling out purchases that you can – and should – live without can be a real damper. Giving up the little things in life can be a difficult adjustment, especially for new parents who are already sacrificing sleep and freedom. For most first-time parents, the financial strain of having a child means looking at where you can cut down on your own expenses. If you fall into this category, this section helps you make some tough choices.

Your fixed costs are food, housing, electricity, heat and transportation. The rest is a mix of choices made by you and your partner about how to live your lives. No hard-and-fast rules exist about what to axe from your life, but depending on your particular needs and your income, the following areas are good places to cut back:

- ✔ **Entertainment:** This category includes the cinema, concerts, cable TV, magazine subscriptions, music, books, DVDs, hobbies, sporting events, and so on. With baby occupying most of your free time, time constraints will help you cut back on sporting events, films and concerts anyway. And instead of spending money on some of the other items, join your local library; as well as books, most have extensive DVD and CD collections. Borrow films from your friends, too, or host a film night and share in the rental and food expenses.

- ✔ **Food:** Whether you eat out often, always dine in or regularly grab coffee, you can make a change in your food spending. Look at your past expenses and find places to save. Even choosing to eat out one less time each month or spending £10 less per week at the supermarket will create big savings over the long haul.

To replace the fun of eating out, host a dinner party or start a rotating dinner club with a group of friends. Assign each attendant a different course so you can drink and dine in style at a fraction of the cost.

- ✔ **Luxury:** New clothing, spa visits, hair care, skin-care products and new jewellery are a few items that can be downgraded, reduced or perhaps axed altogether.

- ✔ **Interest rates:** If you have high interest rates, you're essentially spending money on nothing – clearly a spending habit you won't mind changing! Remortgaging your home on a better deal can save you a bundle in the long run, and if you have a good credit history, try to negotiate a better interest rate with your credit card company. It's not always easy or possible, but it's always worth a call to find out if – and how – you can save.

Create a budget (and stick to it)

After you put your expenses under the microscope and find places to cut back, make a plan and stick to it. Knowing what you plan to spend each month allows you to explore saving options, such as setting up a university account for your baby. Saving money can be a fun game. The more you save, the more thrilling it becomes to push yourself further and watch your personal worth rise.

 If you find yourselves struggling to spend only what you have designated for each item in your monthly budget, use cash. If you take £100 to the supermarket, you have exactly that much to spend. Calculating what you can buy takes more time, but before long you'll be able to quickly recognise what you can and can't afford.

To make a budget, start by breaking down your finances into the following categories, placing a monthly spending allotment next to each:

- Mortgage/rent
- Home/rental insurance
- Electricity
- Gas
- Cable TV
- Water, rates and council tax
- Phone
- Internet
- Home maintenance
- Car payment, insurance and petrol
- Childcare
- Groceries
- Entertainment

Many excellent software programs, books and websites can help you make and maintain a monthly budget. QuickBooks is one of the most popular computer programs for managing your personal finances and even paying your taxes. For the *Dummy*-phile, check out *Personal Finance and Investing All-in-One For Dummies* (Wiley) for everything you need to know to get your finances in order.

Pay off your debt

Not all debt is equally bad. Some debt, such as student loans, tends to have low interest rates and builds future value. Bad debt is anything with a high interest rate; mainly credit cards, and especially credit cards used to purchase unnecessary or disposable goods and subsequently not paid off every month.

Pay off your high-interest debt first, which is probably your credit card bills, and do so as aggressively as your finances allow. Don't use your cards until all of your debt is paid off and after that, only use your card for emergencies and essential expenses, such as groceries. Using it for limited, essential items (that you've budgeted for) will ensure that you can pay off the balance every month. Pay for non-essential items with cash, or you'll end up paying even more for them if you don't pay off your balance each month.

After your credit cards are paid off, start paying off your debt with the next highest interest rate, which is probably a car loan. Also, paying one additional mortgage payment every year can take years off the length of your loan. Remember, this isn't about getting rid of debt altogether. Everyone has debt, and it helps build your credit rating. The goal is to get rid of unnecessary and high-interest debt.

Create an emergency fund

An emergency fund can be a lifesaver for a number of reasons. Job loss happens when you least expect it. Family members get sick and require your time and attention. Houses and cars break down all too often. Whatever life throws at you, it's going to cost you some dough. The rule of thumb changes all the time, but most experts advise saving enough money to cover anywhere from 6 to 12 months of expenses.

If you managed to read that and not faint, take heart – most people don't have that much money tucked away, and a lot of people never will. However, you have to start somewhere, and the less you spend, the more you can save. And now that you have a baby to care for, being able to handle the unexpected expenses is more important than ever.

Make a plan that works for you and your family. If it's easier to start a savings account and slowly move over money each month after bills are paid, go for it. For some, having a set amount or percentage of salary automatically moved into an account each month is easiest. To begin saving, try putting 5 per cent of your monthly salary into a separate savings account. If after a few months you find you still have extra money in your current account, start saving more.

Parenting on the cheap

People tell you that babies are expensive, and, for the most part, they're right. All of the things that babies need to survive add up quickly, especially over time, which is why buying only what you need is of the utmost importance.

Baby stuff is cuter and more expensive than ever before, and more and more parents are buying high-end goods. If you don't have the money for the £500 buggy that all of the other parents in your neighbourhood seem to have, don't buy it. Your baby doesn't need – and won't remember having – an expensive cot or buggy, and he certainly doesn't need nicer clothes than you wear.

Create a monthly budget for your baby expenses. Buy the essentials first and use any leftover money to buy secondary items, such as new toys. Babies don't need a lot to play with; in fact, your tot will probably like the packaging the toy came in better than the toy itself.

Buying lightly used goods from nearly new shops will save you a fortune, and, considering that babies grow in and out of clothes, toys and furniture very quickly, you're likely to find exactly what you want at a fraction of the cost. You can also utilise online sites such as eBay and Freecycle to get what you need cheaply or even free!

Set up a retirement account

Taking care of yourself first means ensuring that your kids won't have to in the future. It is vital that new parents begin saving for their own retirement. As your kids grow, so will your financial needs, which means you need to start saving when you're young in order to have enough to live the way you want to when you retire.

Work with a financial advisor

If numbers make your head spin or if you're not sure that you have the right kind or enough of the savings, insurance and retirement accounts you need to support your lifestyle, you may benefit from working with a financial advisor. Consultations are usually either on a fixed fee basis or on commission from sales (of life insurance, investments, and so on).

If your advisor is unnecessarily pressurising you into buying his company's wares, beware. His main role is to help you prosper financially, and if you're not interested in or in a position to buy something he's pushing, seek advice from someone else. Yes, he has a job to do, but don't get duped into signing up for something you don't want. Always take a day or two to think about a financial advisor's advice before committing to anything and, when possible, seek a second opinion.

Mind your credit rating

If the only ratings you keep track of involve Hollywood blockbusters, you're probably long overdue for a check of your credit rating. Your credit rating changes all the time, so periodically check to make sure you're on track and your credit history has no mistakes. Your credit rating affects the interest rates of every line of credit you have, and a mistake may be costing you on your mortgage, car loan and credit cards.

Credit ratings range from 350 to 850. A very low credit rating is any number below 600. An average credit rating is between about 650 and 700. An excellent credit rating is anything above 700. Your credit rating is reported by three different agencies that provide three different scores. Checking all three is important so that you can clear up any mistakes. You can request your free credit rating from the following:

www.experian.co.uk

www.creditexpert.co.uk

www.equifax.co.uk

Saving Money for Your Child's Education

Every parent wants his child to get the best education money can buy. Not all parents, however, can afford that education, nor do they want their children to accrue vast amounts of student debt.

If you have the luxury of being able to save some money for your child's education, you can save in a personal investment account – that is, a savings, stock, bond or mutual fund account. These accounts give you more control to add or remove money, and you earn capital gains, interest or dividends. You pay taxes on the income each year you earn it, but these accounts give you more freedom to use the savings when and how you see fit. Depending on what level of access you want your child to have to the money, set it up as a trust that can be accessed with conditions, or simply pay the tuition fees yourself.

For parents looking to save for university, make sure first that you have an emergency fund in place and your own future is secure with retirement savings. Don't prioritise your kids' education above these other crucial savings. After all, you don't want your money tied up in a university savings account if your house burns down, and although there's no such thing as a retirement loan, kids taking out student loans to pay for university is now a fact of life.

Getting the Lowdown on Life Insurance

Purchasing life insurance policies in the event that you or your child dies couldn't be more outside the spirit of happiness that comes along with welcoming of a newborn. However, tragedy can strike in many ways and at any time, and although it's not pleasant to think about, life insurance is a must.

Making sure you and your partner have adequate life insurance

Ensuring your child is well cared for in the event of an emergency means confronting your own mortality as well. Buying life insurance for both you and your partner provides a security policy that will allow your family to continue living the life you're all accustomed to without financial ruin in the event one or both of you were to die. Now that you're a parent, it's your responsibility to make sure that bills can be paid and food can be put on the table – even in the event of your death.

Policy needs vary based on your financial circumstances, but the amount you buy should be enough to cover not just funeral costs, but a few years of your current income and expenses, as well as funds to pay off any debts you currently have. This safety net will keep your family financially sound while they deal with their grief.

Considering a policy for your baby

Buying life insurance for your baby is a controversial and unsavoury topic. Many financial experts say it's a waste of money because a life insurance policy is necessary only when the death of the individual will cause financial stress on a family. For many lower- and middle-income families, however, a policy that would cover the cost of the funeral is well worth the monthly payment.

Whole-life coverage versus term

Not all life insurance policies are the same. Some policies are 'rentals', covering a child through a certain age and then offering no more benefit. If you elect to go the 'buying' route for a policy, it will start your child on the right track to financial security for retirement. You can choose between two basic types of policy that determine the price, coverage level and longevity of the policy:

- **Whole-life coverage:** As the name implies, a whole-life policy stays with your child for his entire life. This permanent insurance has a fixed premium that never increases as your child ages and offers the policy owner a guaranteed cash value against which the owner can borrow money in case of emergency.

   Buying whole-life coverage for your baby usually doesn't require a medical check-up. It is important to speak with a professional before purchasing. You won't be able to cash in the whole-life policy at any time for full value, and depending on your financial situation, saving money in an interest-yielding account may be a better idea. That way, you can always access the money you've invested.

- **Term coverage:** Term insurance is sometimes referred to as a 'rental policy' because the named person on the policy will never own it like one does with whole-life coverage. Think of it as a magazine subscription with huge financial benefits: as long as you have a subscription, you're covered. But when the subscription runs out – the policy expires – you stop getting coverage.

   The money you invest is simply going toward 'what if' protection. The cost is generally a fraction of the price of whole-life coverage, which is why it's such an attractive option for some parents. Plans generally come in 10- to 30-year terms. However, premiums are not fixed and do increase as your baby ages.

How much coverage is enough?

Determining how much coverage you should buy depends on your budget. Buy only what you can afford. The more payout benefit you purchase, the more you pay each month. If you're purchasing term insurance, you don't need to buy a policy that will exceed the costs of a funeral and, perhaps, any wage losses resulting from unpaid leave during your grieving period.

Buy only what you can afford to pay every month. Talk with a financial advisor to determine if a whole-life policy is actually the best investment for your child or if another form of savings would yield bigger rewards for him down the road – and still provide you with a safety net in case of death.

Taking Care of Legal Matters

Arranging legal matters is an important step in ensuring your child's well-being in the case of your early death. As unpleasant as the topic may be, you need to sit down with your partner as soon as possible and make decisions about what will happen to your assets and who will take care of your child if you die, and what should happen if either of you is incapacitated. Then make those decisions legally binding by creating a formal will and establishing power of attorney. These tasks aren't fun, but the peace of mind they give you is worth it.

Although most of the forms you need to make these decisions and declarations are available for free online, the only way to make sure that your forms are valid and written in accordance with the law is to have them reviewed by a solicitor. Paying a solicitor is an added expense, but it's worth the money to know your family will be taken care of in the event you are no longer around.

Creating a will

Drawing up a will doesn't have to be as macabre as reading a Stephen King novel. As a soon-to-be or new parent, having a will can bring you peace of mind by leaving no questions about what will happen to your possessions (and children!) when you die. A will includes three provisions:

- ✔ **Who will inherit the money in your bank accounts, property, vehicles and personal possessions when you die.** Most dads have simple wills that leave everything to their partners and, in the event they both die, to their children.

- ✔ **Who will be your children's guardian in case you and your partner are incapacitated or die.** This is your chance to make sure your child will be cared for by the person of your choice and not a relative you wouldn't choose or foster care.

- ✔ **Who will manage any property and money you leave to your child until he reaches a designated age.** Most people name a single executor of their will who is charged with carrying out their wishes. However, some people are more comfortable having the person responsible for carrying out the will's commands to be separate from the person who controls the money.

A will doesn't trump the beneficiaries listed on life insurance policies. Make sure to contact your life insurance company to make the desired changes to those policies, such as adding your new child as a beneficiary.

Making your will

You don't have to go the solicitor route to make a will. Several do-it-yourself computer programs and books (such as *Wills, Probate and Inheritance Tax For Dummies* [Wiley]) provide simple step-by-step instructions for arranging what happens after you die.

Filling in the blanks and hitting print doesn't automatically offer you the protection you need. Any will not made with a solicitor still has to be authorised in order to be valid in the eyes of the law. Most people have a copy of their will residing with their solicitor who drew it up for them.

Make a separate will for each parent. A joint will is binding after the death of even one person, and that makes it difficult for the surviving parent to make changes that may better suit his changed circumstances. Separate wills are especially important when children are involved, because finances change and you want your partner to have access to funds in order to care for your kids. Name your spouse or partner as the sole beneficiary to ensure that she has 100 per cent control of your assets, and have concrete, detailed discussions about how you want the dispersing of money and property, as well as your funeral and burial, handled in the event of your untimely demise.

Appointing guardians

If you have children, guardianship should be addressed when you create a will. If you work with a solicitor, he'll be able to help you fill out all the necessary paperwork. However, if you use an online form or a software program, be sure that it includes the appropriate forms.

If you're unsure of the legal requirements, consult your solicitor. Most forms require a signature from both parents and the appointed guardian as well as legal authorisation.

A will allows you to designate temporary guardianship in the case that your named guardian lives a long way away or can't come for your child immediately. This temporary situation will keep your child out of temporary foster care and in the loving home of your choice.

Guardianship is a huge responsibility for the person you ask. When approaching him, keep in mind that you may not get an immediate yes. In fact, if the person you ask needs some time to think it over, it's a good sign that he understands the responsibility and won't make rash decisions he may later regret. This person will not only be in charge of your child but will also have to cover any of the financial gaps not covered by the money you set aside to be used for your child's upbringing.

Questions to ask yourself when choosing a legal guardian or godparent

When deciding who would make the best guardian for your child in case of your death, consider the following questions:

✔ Does the person love my child?

✔ Is the person good with children in general?

✔ How important is it that my child's guardian be a family member?

✔ Will my child be uprooted from his home to move in with the guardian?

✔ Does the person have the same parenting philosophies as me?

✔ Is the person going to raise my child with the same religious beliefs?

✔ Does the person have any medical conditions that would prevent him from being a long-term, able-bodied guardian?

✔ Will my child create too much of a personal, professional or financial strain for the person?

✔ Does the person have a stable home life and career?

✔ Will this person guarantee my child has access to his family?

✔ Does this person value the same things I do (education, music, community, and so on)?

If the person you ask declines, ask for more information about why he refused. Perhaps you have information that can assuage any fears he may have about the job. However, if the person you ask (even after further discussion) isn't up for the job, find someone else. Yes, it will be disappointing, but respect that person's honesty and forthrightness in admitting he is the wrong person for the job. And when it comes down to it, finding the right person is most important.

Appointing an executor

The person you appoint as executor is in charge of *executing* your will, or making sure that taxes and debts are paid and your estate is distributed according to your will. Avoid appointing someone as an executor who is also a beneficiary of your will. You can name co-executors if you want one person to manage your money and the other to manage, say, your property. It can be good to utilise different people's skills and it gives you back-up if one person drops the ball.

You designate an executor using the same online or software program you use to make a will, or when creating a will with your solicitor. Make sure that the person you designate is willing and able to perform the role. Most forms that designate an executor for your will require you to provide one or two contingency executors in case the first named executor cannot perform the job.

When there's no will

If you die without having made a will (intestate), the estate is then distributed according to the laws of intestacy. A set of statutory rules apply that leave a person's estate to their next of kin in a fixed order. However, this course of action is not to be recommended!

Establishing power of attorney

Granting power of attorney to someone gives that person the power to make decisions – both legal and medical – in the event that you're incapacitated. The person you name will be able to make important decisions about life support and control of your bank accounts.

Generally included as part of the will-making process, appointing power of attorney takes only a simple form that usually must be signed by you and the named power of attorney and then authorised.

Experts suggest choosing someone you trust but who isn't a close friend or family member. After all, even if you've made it clear that you don't want to be on life support for an extended period of time, your mother may have difficulty pulling the plug. Select a person who you can trust to follow through with your wishes.

The power of attorney should follow what you outline in your will, so go over your will with that person to make sure he's comfortable following your orders. If not, find someone else, or complications may arise that will cause added stress for everyone involved. What's most important is finding a person you can trust who will be informed about your wishes and make sure they're followed.

Part V
The Part of Tens

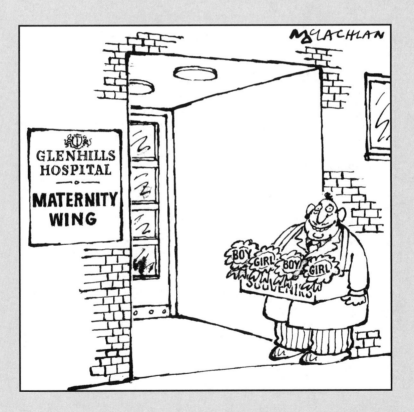

In this part...

The Part of Tens provides practical tips on everything- from reading your partner's mind to being a super dad. We also look at the wonderful world of stay-at-home fatherhood, should you be considering that increasingly-common route.

Chapter 16

Ten Things She Won't Ask for but Will Expect

. . . .

In This Chapter

▶ Showing your excitement about being a father

▶ Helping your partner with emotional and physical support

. . . .

During the course of your partner's pregnancy – and many months thereafter – she'll expect myriad tasks, words of comfort and loving gestures from you without her having to ask for what she wants. Sadly, you weren't born with advanced psychic aptitude, and therefore you'll have to infer a few *musts* to keep peace around the house.

Follow these ten simple tips to make sure your partner gets everything she needs.

Keep It Complimentary

Face it – you'll never know what it's like to give up your body so that someone else can grow inside of you. That said, it probably isn't too hard to remember the last time you got a new haircut or lost ten pounds and then waited around for someone to tell you how nice you looked.

Going fishing for compliments is never a fun or fruitful excursion, so try to spare your partner from going to that length. When her hormones and ever-increasing waistline are waging a fully-fledged attack on her insecurities, remind her early and often exactly how beautiful she looks. And the best part is, you won't have to lie. It may be hard to imagine finding your partner gorgeous when she's carrying around 30 to 40 extra pounds, but pregnant women glow, and knowing that your partner is having your baby will make her extremely attractive.

When she asks you how she looks or if she's got fat (and she will ask you!), flatter her no end, deny it vehemently and thank her for her sacrifices.

Start a Baby Book

Baby books, with their endless pages of blank space calling out for someone to fill in the missing data, can be a daunting undertaking, especially when chronicling the journey is left solely to the mum-to-be/new mummy. Most women won't admit it, but during pregnancy they're looking for constant signs that you're just as committed to bringing up a child together as she is. Filling out a baby book together can be the perfect way to put into words just how ready you are for baby.

A great way to exhibit your commitment to and excitement about the baby is to buy a baby book that reflects your personalities. If you and the mum-to-be are the journal types, pick one that offers lots of space to write about how you're feeling during each trimester and your thoughts about becoming a parent. If you fall into the less-is-more crowd, choose a book that adheres to a mostly fill-in-the-blank format. Many themed books are available, running the gamut from religious to hipster chic, so choose one that represents both parents.

The baby book is a time-honoured time capsule that chronicles the pregnancy and early days of your baby's life, and it should be something fun to put together as a couple. Someday that book will mean the world to your child, so make sure to buy one that you'll realistically finish.

Disguise Fitness as Fun

Exercise is of the utmost importance to both baby and mummy, but try telling your partner to get up off the sofa and go for a walk without having something hard thrown at your head. Getting a loved one involved in exercise is never easy to do without hurt feelings, so instead of telling her that she needs to exercise, help her keep fit without making it personal.

Turn fitness into a social activity: plan walks with friends and family or schedule errands together that require you to get up and move around. Plan a treasure hunt to local baby shops to check out the latest gear, or even a hunt with a romantic bent. Even a trip to the shopping centre can be good exercise so long as you steer clear of the food counters.

If your partner has a particular interest in a certain type of exercise, give her a free pass as a gift. Be it yoga, spinning or running, most fitness clubs or personal trainers offer antenatal versions of their classes. Many classes welcome partners, too, and by making it a couples' affair it won't send the message that you think she's fat.

Curb Your Advice

Never has there been a better time to let go of your desire to be right at all costs than now, even if you really *do* know best. Let your partner complain about her job, her body, the mere fact that she's pregnant or whatever, and don't take her complaints, gripes or outbursts personally. Now, that doesn't give her free rein to be a raving lunatic just because she's pregnant, but don't try to solve her problems with your sage wisdom unless she specifically asks for it. Listen to her and validate what she's feeling, but don't tell her how to fix it.

Also, avoid telling her what to eat, when to exercise, that she needs to sleep more and so on. Instead, lead by example. If you think she should eat more fruit and vegetables, buy more fruit and vegetables. Or better yet, make meals packed with pregnancy power foods. If you think she needs to rest more, ask her to sit down and do a crossword with you. Telling her what to do won't go down well, so don't waste your breath.

Attend Antenatal Appointments

Repeat after us: antenatal appointments aren't just for the mothers. Yes, your partner is carrying the baby, but that baby didn't get there on her own. You're in this together, and if she has to make time in her schedule to attend countless appointments, ultrasounds and tests, so should you. Doing so will demonstrate to her that you're a team in the bringing up of this baby, and you'll be much more excited about the process if you're as involved as your partner.

Childbirth is an empowering experience for both mother and father, and the more appointments you attend, the more knowledgeable you'll be about the entire process. Being an involved father starts long before the baby arrives. In fact, if you plan on being an equal partner in the raising of your child, it won't just happen overnight. You wouldn't play in a darts match without practice, and you shouldn't enter into parenthood without practising the type of dad you want to be.

If your work schedule doesn't allow for you to attend every appointment, go to as many as possible. Follow up with her immediately after each appointment you miss and ask her for a recap. Ask lots of questions; your partner will be grateful to know you care. Many important decisions and discussions occur during antenatal visits, and even if you can't be present, make sure you remain part of the discussion.

Plan a Getaway

After baby arrives it won't be easy to abandon ship and head for the hills when you need a relaxing reprieve from life. And as the long wait for baby drags on and you both begin to realise how much is going to change in your personal lives after she comes, you may find yourselves looking for one last couples retreat.

Take the lead and plan a trip. Keep in mind that the later your partner is in her pregnancy, the closer to home you'll want to be in case she goes into labour. Also, her body (and especially her bladder) won't be up for sitting on a plane or in the car for long periods of time. Wherever you go, make the trip romantic, personal and quiet. Make it a time to focus on your relationship – just the two of you – because it won't be the focus of your lives for some time to come.

If you plan something during the third trimester, keep in mind that many airlines have restrictions about how close to her due date your partner can travel. Check with your airline before booking tickets, because many require a doctor's note.

Sign Up for an Antenatal Parenting Class

The days of antenatal parenting classes that focus solely on breathing and birthing techniques are over. Today's classes offer opportunities for parents-to-be to explore birthing options, relationships, the type of parents they want to be, first aid and infant care. Find a class that's welcoming to both mother and father and sign up, either through your local hospital or by searching online.

Do Your Homework and Spread the Word

Clearly, if you're reading this book, then you've already done the majority of your homework. Congratulations – you're going to be a great dad. Now don't be afraid to blow your own trumpet. Not every dad-to-be is as prepared as you, and you deserve credit. Make a point of telling your partner how much you've found out in these pages. Ask her, 'Did you know . . . ?' and 'Have you thought about . . . ?' Who knows, you just may teach her something she didn't know. And is there any better feeling in the world than feeling accomplished?

At the very least, you'll set a good example of your own involvement in the future of your relationship. In the past, fathers weren't expected to know anything about pregnancy, and it wasn't all that long ago that the majority of men stayed out of the delivery room and returned to work the day after delivery. The more you know, the more your partner will trust you to care for the baby. Trust is earned, and by educating yourself about babies, you're earning the trust that many fathers of the past forfeited.

Learn Antenatal Massage

Pregnancy puts stress on all the body's joints and ligaments as muscles (and even bones!) shift and expand, causing mothers-to-be to walk, stand, sit and sleep in ways that often are at odds with their normal movements and positions. Add an additional 30 to 40 pounds hanging off her front, and it's no wonder that your average pregnant woman gets achy, tired and downright sore.

Learning the basics of massage can help you help your partner to alleviate many of those aches and pains – and will make you her hero after a long day of carrying around your child. Some hospitals offer antenatal massage classes so ask if these are available in your area. While you're at it, consider learning the ins and outs of infant massage. Research shows that infant massage can help babies digest food and sleep better, and helps prevent and treat colic. Check with your hospital or midwife for more information.

Clean High and Low

The closer you get to delivery time, the more likely your partner is to desire a clean, tidy home. Limited by a rather large belly and an unrelenting tiredness, your partner won't always feel like cleaning or be able to do it. Areas that fall below your partner's knee level and things out of her reach are particularly difficult for her during the latter stages of pregnancy.

But her limitations don't mean that you have to clean everything all by yourself. In fact, the exercise involved in cleaning can be beneficial for her. However, assign yourself the job of picking up everything from the floor on a frequent basis. Clutter-free floors and walkways will prevent her from falling and will keep her from pulling a muscle in her back trying to reach down.

While you're down there, you have a good view of what baby will see when she's crawling around your home. You can always begin baby-proofing your abode; the extra time you give yourself will let you get used to the new limitations and restrictions.

Though it's a myth that a pregnant woman will strangle the baby if she raises her arms above her head, it may be a rather uncomfortable experience. Take the lead on cleaning the blinds, putting away dishes in the cupboards, changing light bulbs and dusting.

Chapter 17

Ten Ways to Be a Super Dad from Day One

*W*hen it comes to parenting, what you don't know won't kill you, but it sure can keep you from making the most of the greatest, most joyous time in your life. After almost a year of waiting for baby to arrive, don't forget that now is the time to have fun. Yes, bringing a teeny, tiny baby into your home evokes a great deal of worrying, but babies aren't as fragile as you may think. If you want to be a super dad, try to follow these tips on how to be a confident, loving and cool father from day one.

Overcome Fragility Fears

Animals can sense fear, and when they know you're afraid, they exploit your weakness at every turn. The same goes for babies, albeit without the evil ulterior motive. If you're afraid of holding your baby, you probably aren't providing a solid, sturdy base for him, and he'll fuss and cry until somebody who is confident takes over the reins. The same holds true for changing nappies, feeding and cuddling.

Repeat after us: I am not going to break my baby. He's designed to survive a first-time parent like yourself, and as long as you're not trying to juggle knives while burping him, chances are that you're both going to be just fine. Babies are small, but so long as you take reasonable safety precautions like never leaving him unattended, always securing him in a car seat and listening closely to the baby monitor during sleep time, you aren't going to hurt him.

The most important tip is to take deep, steady breaths and hold your baby in the same casual-yet-protective way you grasp your iPad. Don't fumble with the baby as you lift him up onto your shoulder. Use firm, fluid movements. The more you act like you know what you're doing, the more the baby will like what you're doing.

Trust Your Instincts

Because babies are designed to be cared for by people who don't have any education in the raising of children, you have no choice but to follow your instincts. Babies have been around since, well, the dawn of man, and all the parents since that time have raised them their own way. It wasn't all that long ago that parents and parents-to-be told stories of their experiences around the campfire instead of relying on modern inventions such as parenting classes and the Internet. We're born with the instinct to care for our children, and so long as you don't have mental or emotional impediments (such as postnatal depression), you'll just know what to do.

Just remember that nobody can know your baby better than you do, and despite the seeming lack of faith others may show toward your judgement (how warmly you dress him, how often you feed him, how you hold him and so on), the only truly vital task of the parent is to ensure safety. Trust yourself, educate yourself and you'll not steer that little one wrong.

Bond Skin-to-Skin, Eye-to-Eye

Mothers get an amazing opportunity to spend skin-to-skin time with baby while breastfeeding. This sensory bond is so important that mere moments after the baby is born, the midwife will often place him on mum's bare chest. Studies show that skin-to-skin contact increases the bond that both mother and child feel, as well as the soothing feeling babies experience from listening to mum's heartbeat. Also, a newborn's eyesight is just powerful enough to see the distance from the breast to mum's eyes.

You won't be breastfeeding, so you have far fewer opportunities to experience the same closeness. Yes, baby's head will rest on your hands and arms, and you can get close and make eye contact, but that doesn't provide the same bonded feeling. When baby is only in his nappy, take off your shirt and place him on your chest. It may sound a little cheesy, but it's an important bonding experience for fathers as well as mothers, and it gives you and baby the opportunity to meet skin-to-skin and eye-to-eye for the first time.

Manage Frustrations

Admit it – your baby is the most beautiful sight you've ever seen. As you stare into the wondering eyes of your newborn you may think it impossible to ever feel anything but absolute adoration for this child. However, babies often are exhausting and unmanageable beings who wake you up in the middle of the night, cry endlessly without giving you a clue as to what's wrong and require 100 per cent of your attention.

Feeling frustrated is okay, because parenting, especially when you're brand new at it, can and will be a frustrating experience from time to time. In preparation for when that cute bundle of joy becomes an obstinate teen, here are some simple ways to manage your frustration:

- ✔ **Control the controllable.** It's easier said than done, but some things you can change and some things you can't. Babies do not sleep through the night. Babies spit up. Babies cry for no good reason. Don't waste your time trying to solve problems that aren't really problems. As long as you are sure he's not unwell, if your baby has a clean nappy, a full belly and a wind-free stomach, yet still continues to fuss, just put on some noise-cancelling headphones and let him cry. Unless something is wrong, don't worry about him.

- ✔ **Monitor baby's routine.** Keep a log of when baby sleeps, wakes, eats, poos and pees. Understanding his routine takes a lot of the guesswork out of determining what he needs at any given time. If you discover that your little one starts getting fussy after being awake for 90 minutes, you'll know how to structure your day to make sure that everyone – including you – gets what they need to function.

- ✔ **Blow off steam.** Pick your poison – running, playing computer games, listening to music, reading – whatever it is that puts your mind at ease, and make sure you take time to continue engaging in it. If you find yourself getting frustrated, spend five minutes doing your favourite activity. Even a walk around the block can be a great way to hit your reset button.

- ✔ **Lean on your support system.** When the going gets tough and you feel like you need to get out of town, do it! Call a babysitter, a friend or a family member to fill in for you, even if it's just for an hour so you can run to the shops in peace. Don't discount the benefits of time alone or with your partner to make your frustrations dissipate.

✔ **Sleep in shifts.** Sleep is a hot commodity among the parenting set, and before long you'll be coveting every available minute of shut-eye. However, if baby is constantly waking during the night, both you and your partner will quickly lose patience in the wee hours of the morning. Though it's not the ideal situation, try taking turns sleeping for blocks of time in the night and throughout the day while on leave (or the weekends). You need to get as much sleep as possible, even if those hours aren't consecutive. The key to keeping your frustrations in check just may be two hours of peaceful slumber.

Embrace Your Silly Side

By now you've probably made a list of all the things you're not going to do as a parent. For many too-cool-for-school dads, that list includes such things as baby talk, funny faces and the pure lunacy of dressing up, tea parties and dancing that requires dads to abandon traditional masculinity at the door in favour of fun.

Do all the things on that list. Don't feel stupid and don't feel restrained by how you think men should behave. Babies (and kids, for that matter) love expressive faces, singing and daft voices, and while acting silly may leave you in a shroud of self-consciousness, you'll get over it the instant your baby laughs or smiles at your mad antics. Allow yourself to have fun, and you'll reap the rewards for life.

Get Out

Going to work doesn't qualify as getting out of the house. Yes, it may be a nice change of pace to spend time doing things that don't require baby wipes, but the kind of getting out you need is of the date variety.

You may be surprised to know that getting out of the house is easier when your baby is younger. Make sure to schedule a date within the first month of baby's arrival. Start slowly – new mums (and many dads) find it hard to leave baby for the first time. Ask a trusted friend or family member to watch baby while you grab a quick bite to eat at your favourite restaurant.

Ground rules? Don't talk about baby. You may not achieve this almost impossible goal, but shoot for the stars. You need to connect as adults again, not just as parents, and that brief time away will remind you why you love your partner so much. And, upon returning home, you'll have a welcome reminder of just how much you love that baby.

Teach Baby New Tricks

You may think babies discover the world of their own volition, but the truth is that you need to give your little one a push. In fact, the more time you put into teaching and nurturing your baby, the prouder you'll be when he learns to roll over, clap, wave bye-bye or play with a toy. Bonding happens daily with babies, and a child's way of thinking is practically set in stone by age 3. You can have a huge influence on the rate at which your child develops, but more importantly, you can have a huge influence on your child's entire life by getting involved in playtime and the open expression of love.

Following are some milestones you can help baby achieve in the first six months:

- ✓ **Tracking objects:** Slowly move a colourful object back and forth and up and down in front of baby's eyes. This activity helps the brain begin to follow movement. Sound tracking can also be done in the same way.

- ✓ **Making sounds:** Your baby makes a lot of strange sounds, and a supremely important part of language development is hearing you repeat those sounds back to him. Babies have their own language that you don't understand, and the more they hear it the more they'll talk, which aids in language development down the road.

- ✓ **Reaching and grabbing:** Dangle colourful toys and baby-safe objects in front of your child and wait for him to reach for them. Encourage gripping by wrapping baby's hand around the object and letting go.

- ✓ **Peek-a-boo:** Babies will laugh as you disappear and reappear time and again, all while beginning to understand the idea of cause and effect. Showing baby the mirror is also a fun, mind-expanding game.

- ✓ **Rolling over:** Lay your baby on his back on a play mat or a colourful rug to encourage him to turn over and begin to explore. When he can support his own head, give him plenty of tummy time on his belly, which develops the stomach muscles and allows him to roll over.

- ✓ **Crawling:** New studies show that the way babies' brains react during crawling (the right brain controls the left side of the body and vice versa) is an important milestone that can help reduce behavioural and mental disorders in children. Help ensure your child can crawl by putting a coveted toy just out of reach and waiting for him to come and get it.

Rough and Tumble the Safe Way

Though we don't want to engage in gender stereotyping, fathers are often more likely to get physical during playtime with their kids. And although you probably won't be wrestling with your newborn (please, don't wrestle your newborn!), go ahead and swing him in your arms, hold him up high over your head, rub your scratchy face into his belly, tickle him and chew on his feet. Mum may think it's too much, but more than likely, baby will think it's hysterical. As long as you're being safe, have fun.

Read Aloud . . . and Not Just from Baby Books

Read to baby every single day. Not only will he love the sound of your voice, but he'll also learn to speak from hearing the constant repetition of speech patterns. And the more you read to baby, the more likely it is that he'll develop a wide vocabulary and the ability to speak at a younger age.

While baby is too young to truly enjoy kids' books, don't be afraid to read him passages from the novels you want to read. It's a good way to engage in adult activities while also helping your baby grow smarter every day.

Send Mum Away

Unless you're fortunate enough to be a work-at-home dad, you'll need to make sure that you block off some one-to-one time with your baby. Finding your own way as a parent and learning that you are capable, are important steps in feeling empowered as a new dad. Which means that mum needs to go away for a while.

Book an appointment at the spa for your partner and spend the afternoon doing everyday activities with baby. Take him for a walk, feed him, change him or even go out to the coffee shop and read the paper with him. Regardless of the activities you do together, this time establishes one-to-one intimacy with your child and proves to yourself and your partner that you are capable of taking care of your child on your own.

Chapter 18

Ten Musts for the Stay-at-Home Dad

*M*ore and more dads are making the decision to leave the workplace behind to stay at home and take care of their children. Whether you're leaving the workforce altogether or balancing work with childcare responsibilities, it's important that both you and your partner acknowledge that bringing up a child is a job. And although you aren't pocketing a pay packet to look after your little one, managing your new role as you would a traditional career will keep you from pulling out your hair and feeling underappreciated.

In fact, now that you're working in the home, you need to treat your home like your workplace. Employ the ten essential tips in this chapter to keep your new business running smoothly.

Practise Hands-Free Parenting

One thing you take for granted when working at an office job is the presence of two empty hands at your disposal. At work, balancing a coffee mug and a telephone may constitute multitasking. When staying at home with baby, however, you'll find yourself with a shortage of hands to complete the myriad tasks you attempt during the course of any given day. Just the act of making coffee can be a challenge some days.

Multitasking takes on a whole new meaning when you're home alone with baby, especially while baby is awake and in constant need of your attention. Using some of the following contraptions makes it possible for you to do something else while still providing loving, excellent care for baby:

- ✔ **Front baby carriers:** They aren't just good for walks and shopping – you can use one while you play a game on the Wii, do chores or even walk around the house reading if your baby is windy and needs constant movement. Just make sure not to do anything dangerous, like chopping vegetables, and don't whack the baby in the head with the Wii controller.

- ✔ **Play mat with dangling toys:** Baby is entertained by dangling animals, mirrors and flashing lights while dad gets the chance to do other things. It can also be used to give baby some much-needed tummy time, which encourages crawling.

- ✔ **Bouncy chair:** You can bounce this with one foot to keep babies who always want to jiggle happy.

- ✔ **Playpen:** This enclosed area provides baby with a safe place to move around while you move around. It gives you the peace of mind that she's contained in an area where she won't get hurt. It's a great solution for people with pets, especially rambunctious or overly loving pets, and it protects the pets from the baby, too.

- ✔ **Swing or doorway bouncer:** For a baby who can hold her head up and loves to bounce, a swing or bouncer is endless entertainment and frees you to move around the house.

Much like you would at the gym, put baby on the circuit-training programme. Moving her from place to place helps her develop new muscles, provides different views and gives you as much peace as possible before she starts screaming, pooing or eating.

Start a Habits Log

Babies, like adults, aren't 100 per cent consistent about what times they eat, sleep, poo and play every single day. Chances are, however, that your baby has developed (and will continue to develop) some distinct patterns that you may not have picked up on. Understanding these patterns can help you plan your day and make it possible for you to be as productive as possible.

In a standard notebook, write down what your baby does through-out the day, including the start and end times. For bottles, keep track of how many ounces she drank. Knowing how much time baby generally goes between naps – and how long she naps at different times in the day – makes it easier for you to plan when you can get out, when you can make a phone call or when you can relax.

Keeping a log also helps you understand what your baby may be crying about, which makes your life a lot less stressful! If she typically naps every 90 minutes and drinks a bottle every three hours, you can consult your log to get a good idea of what she may need.

Develop a Nap Routine

Babies can't control when they're tired, which means you probably won't be able to put your child down for a nap at the exact same time every day, at least not in the early months. That said, you do need to put your child down in the same way every single day.

Develop sleepy-time cues, such as turning out the lights and turning on soft music, to let your baby know that it's time to settle down for sleep. Even playing the same song (or singing the same song) every time before you put her down helps her learn to expect what's coming. Creating this routine makes the naptime process run more smoothly and cuts down on the amount of time it takes to put baby to sleep.

Walk and Talk

Especially for the father who chooses to continue having an outside job in addition to watching the baby, 'mobile meetings' are essential. Talking on the phone with a baby in the house, especially for business purposes, can be one of the more challenging aspects. Concentrating is hard – and your professionalism is compromised – if a screaming baby is audible during your phone calls.

If you live in a quiet area, you may want to talk on the phone while pushing a buggy around the neighbourhood. Most kids are calmed by the great outdoors and the movement of the buggy, or even time in the front carrier, can allow you to talk in peace.

If you've been holding out on purchasing a Bluetooth, now's the time to buy. As described in the 'Practise Hands-Free Parenting' section, you'll have better things to do with your hands than hold a phone. Also, liberal use of the mute button when you aren't speaking is highly recommended. When you walk in public, cancelling out the noise from traffic, wind and other people is polite to the person on the other end and keeps unexpected baby outbursts from interrupting the conversation as much as possible.

If walking while talking isn't possible and you must stay indoors, use the mute button, and if the baby is making a fuss when you need to speak, there's no shame in putting her in her cot, shutting the door and stepping out into the hallway for a minute. Babies cry, and as long as you don't put anything sharp or dangerous in the cot, she'll be fine for a short time while you conduct your business.

Get Your Music On

One of the most amazing things about infants is that they come out ready to adapt, mimic and adore everything you love. Most babies will find music calming and funny, and it can teach them about cause and effect. If you play an instrument, make music time a part of your day from the outset. Not only will it be a bond between you and your child that will last a lifetime, but it will also probably pacify and amuse, which is what every stay-at-home dad strives to achieve.

If you're not musically inclined, even turning on your favourite music and clapping, whistling or humming along can do the trick. And when baby begins to explore objects, she'll begin to see the musical possibilities in everything, and you can take all the credit. Music has been shown to increase cognitive development in babies, so even playing her toy xylophone has benefits.

Kids don't need to be exposed to children's music until they're able to ask for it to be played. Whether you're a classic rock guy or an indie-music hipster, play what you like and wait with bated breath for the day your baby begins responding to her – your – favourite songs.

Nurture Independence

Just because looking out for your child is your job doesn't mean you should hold, rock, walk or play with her every hour of every day. In fact, the more frequently you give your child the chance to be independent, the sooner you'll find more independence during your daytime hours.

Utilise safe items such as her playpen, cot, bouncy chair and so on and feel free to move about your house within earshot of your child. If she gets too used to being in the same room with you and being able to see you at all times, putting her down for a nap, leaving her with a babysitter or even going to the bathroom will all be more difficult.

Relax When You Can

While at your old job, at times you may have felt the need to surf the Internet for a few minutes to unwind after a hard morning, or maybe you even took the entire day off to relax because you just didn't feel like working. As the stay-at-home dad, you won't always have the option to take time for yourself when you just feel like blowing off steam, and you certainly can't decide on a whim to take a day off.

Utilise at least one naptime to its fullest extent by doing whatever activity helps you recharge your batteries and feel refreshed. Maybe it's a shower, or maybe it's a nap of your own. Or maybe it's reclaiming that lost time of Internet mindlessness. Don't spend every naptime cleaning or rushing around to finish up those last bits of work, because everyone deserves a break. Allow yourself the same opportunity you would at any job – cut yourself some slack and regroup.

Personalise Your Business

For the dads who continue to do outside work, keeping your day-time set-up a secret can be a disaster. Be proud of what you're doing and be honest with the people you work with. Make sure to schedule meetings, phone calls and deadlines to suit the schedules of all people involved, and be honest about why you need to meet when you do. The support you get from people when you tell them that you're working from home to take care of your child can be both surprising and moving. Embracing your new role and personalising your business around it can buy you patience and flexibility from others.

Secure a Daytime Support System

If you think you can go it alone, you're wrong. That's not to say that you won't be able to manage well enough by yourself on the average day, but times will come when you're unwell, have a meeting or just need a break. Don't wait until the need arises to have help on-call that can come in to relieve you as needed.

 Rely on a mix of babysitters, friends, family members and other stay-at-home parents in your neighbourhood. To keep costs down, consider trading favours with other parents in your neighbourhood – just keep in mind that this arrangement means you'll be saddled with their kids at some point, too. This support system is also a good idea for the night-time, allowing you and your partner to go on a date every once in a while.

Even if you have a family member just up the road who's always ready to lend a hand, getting your kid familiar with a variety of people is a good idea just in case your relative isn't available to pitch in. No matter whom you choose, make sure that both you and your partner are comfortable with that person as well as her home set-up if you drop off your child there.

Plan Lunches

Invest time each weekend to plan and prepare meals ahead of time, or you may find yourself making unhealthy choices – financially and calorifically – during the weekdays. Parenting requires a lot of energy and time, and if you don't have food that's ready to eat at your disposal, you're more likely to pick up fast food, eat a chocolate bar instead of a meal or skip meals altogether.

Make sure to prepare healthy meals full of protein, vegetables and whole grains, which will give you a boost of energy for the afternoon. Also, keep on hand high-protein, natural snacks, such as nuts, fruit and cereal bars, which can serve as pick-me-ups for the late-day grind.

Index

Notes

Notes

Notes

FOR DUMMIES®

Making Everything Easier! ™

UK editions

BUSINESS

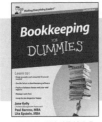

978-0-470-97626-5

978-0-470-97211-3

978-0-470-71119-4

REFERENCE

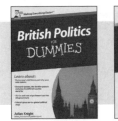

978-0-470-68637-9

978-0-470-97450-6

978-0-470-74535-9

HOBBIES

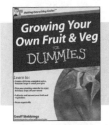

978-0-470-69960-7

978-0-470-68641-6

978-0-470-68178-7

Asperger's Syndrome For Dummies
978-0-470-66087-4

Boosting Self-Esteem For Dummies
978-0-470-74193-1

British Sign Language
For Dummies
978-0-470-69477-0

Coaching with NLP For Dummies
978-0-470-97226-7

Cricket For Dummies
978-0-470-03454-5

Diabetes For Dummies, 3rd Edition
978-0-470-97711-8

English Grammar For Dummies
978-0-470-05752-0

Flirting For Dummies
978-0-470-74259-4

Football For Dummies
978-0-470-68837-3

IBS For Dummies
978-0-470-51737-6

Improving Your Relationship
For Dummies
978-0-470-68472-6

Lean Six Sigma For Dummies
978-0-470-75626-3

Life Coaching For Dummies,
2nd Edition
978-0-470-66554-1

Management For Dummies,
2nd Edition
978-0-470-97769-9

Nutrition For Dummies, 2nd Edition
978-0-470-97276-2

**Available wherever books are sold. For more information or to order direct go to
www.wiley.com or call +44 (0) 1243 843291**

30093 (p1)

FOR DUMMIES®

A world of resources to help you grow

UK editions

SELF—HELP

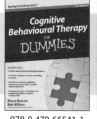

978-0-470-66541-1

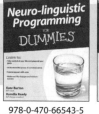

978-0-470-66543-5

978-0-470-66086-7

STUDENTS

978-0-470-68820-5

978-0-470-74711-7

978-1-119-99134-2

HISTORY

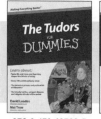

978-0-470-68792-5

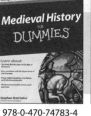

978-0-470-74783-4

978-0-470-97819-1

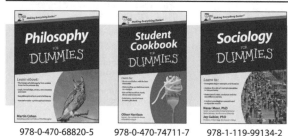

Origami Kit For Dummies
978-0-470-75857-1

Overcoming Depression For Dummies
978-0-470-69430-5

Positive Psychology For Dummies
978-0-470-72136-0

PRINCE2 For Dummies, 2009 Edition
978-0-470-71025-8

Psychometric Tests For Dummies
978-0-470-75366-8

Reading the Financial Pages
For Dummies
978-0-470-71432-4

Rugby Union For Dummies, 3rd Edition
978-1-119-99092-5

Sage 50 Accounts For Dummies
978-0-470-71558-1

Self-Hypnosis For Dummies
978-0-470-66073-7

Starting a Business For Dummies,
3rd Edition
978-0-470-97810-8

Study Skills For Dummies
978-0-470-74047-7

Teaching English as a Foreign Language
For Dummies
978-0-470-74576-2

Time Management For Dummies
978-0-470-77765-7

Training Your Brain For Dummies
978-0-470-97449-0

Work-Life Balance For Dummies
978-0-470-71380-8

Writing a Dissertation For Dummies
978-0-470-74270-9

**Available wherever books are sold. For more information or to order direct go to
www.wiley.com or call +44 (0) 1243 843291**

30093 (p2)

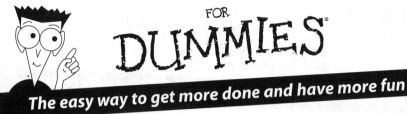

FOR DUMMIES®

The easy way to get more done and have more fun

LANGUAGES

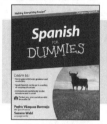

Spanish
978-0-470-68815-1
UK Edition

French
978-1-118-00464-7

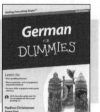

German
978-0-470-90101-4

MUSIC

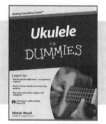

Ukulele
978-0-470-97799-6
UK Edition

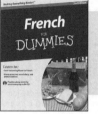

Guitar Chords
978-0-470-66603-6
Lay-flat, UK Edition

DJing
978-0-470-66372-1
UK Edition

SCIENCE & MATHS

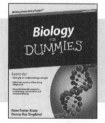

Biology
978-0-470-59875-7

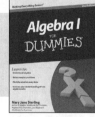

Algebra I
978-0-470-55964-2

Genetics
978-0-470-55174-5

Art For Dummies
978-0-7645-5104-8

Bass Guitar For Dummies, 2nd
Edition
978-0-470-53961-3

Criminology For Dummies
978-0-470-39696-4

Currency Trading For Dummies
978-0-470-12763-6

Drawing For Dummies, 2nd Edition
978-0-470-61842-4

Forensics For Dummies
978-0-7645-5580-0

Guitar For Dummies, 2nd Edition
978-0-7645-9904-0

Index Investing For Dummies
978-0-470-29406-2

Knitting For Dummies, 2nd Edition
978-0-470-28747-7

Music Theory For Dummies
978-0-7645-7838-0

Piano For Dummies, 2nd Edition
978-0-470-49644-2

Physics For Dummies, 2nd Edition
978-0-470-90324-7

Schizophrenia For Dummies
978-0-470-25927-6

Sex For Dummies, 3rd Edition
978-0-470-04523-7

Sherlock Holmes For Dummies
978-0-470-48444-9

Solar Power Your Home
For Dummies, 2nd Edition
978-0-470-59678-4

The Koran For Dummies
978-0-7645-5581-7

Available wherever books are sold. For more information or to order direct go to
www.wiley.com or call +44 (0) 1243 843291

30093 (p3)

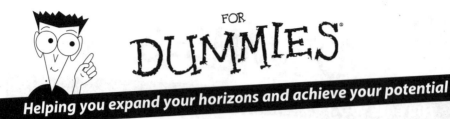

FOR DUMMIES®

Helping you expand your horizons and achieve your potential

COMPUTER BASICS

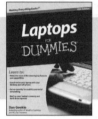

978-0-470-57829-2   978-0-470-46542-4   978-0-470-49743-2

DIGITAL PHOTOGRAPHY

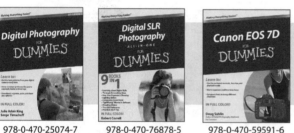

978-0-470-25074-7   978-0-470-76878-5   978-0-470-59591-6

MICROSOFT OFFICE 2010

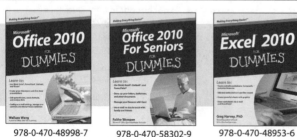

978-0-470-48998-7   978-0-470-58302-9   978-0-470-48953-6

Access 2010 For Dummies
978-0-470-49747-0

Android Application Development
For Dummies
978-0-470-77018-4

AutoCAD 2011 For Dummies
978-0-470-59539-8

C++ For Dummies, 6th Edition
978-0-470-31726-6

Computers For Seniors For Dummies,
2nd Edition
978-0-470-53483-0

Dreamweaver CS5 For Dummies
978-0-470-61076-3

Green IT For Dummies
978-0-470-38688-0

iPad All-in-One For Dummies
978-0-470-92867-7

Macs For Dummies, 11th Edition
978-0-470-87868-2

Mac OS X Snow Leopard For Dummies
978-0-470-43543-4

Photoshop CS5 For Dummies
978-0-470-61078-7

Photoshop Elements 9 For Dummies
978-0-470-87872-9

Search Engine Optimization
For Dummies, 4th Edition
978-0-470-88104-0

The Internet For Dummies,
12th Edition
978-0-470-56095-2

Visual Studio 2010 All-In-One
For Dummies
978-0-470-53943-9

Web Analytics For Dummies
978-0-470-09824-0

Word 2010 For Dummies
978-0-470-48772-3

**Available wherever books are sold. For more information or to order direct go to
www.wiley.com or call +44 (0) 1243 843291**

30093 (p4)